Health and disability

Manual for WHO Disability Assessment Schedule

WHODAS 2.0

Editors

TB Üstün, N Kostanjsek,

S Chatterji, J Rehm

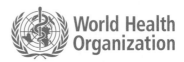

World Health
Organization

WHO Library Cataloguing-in-Publication Data

Measuring Health and Disability: Manual for WHO Disability Assessment Schedule (WHODAS 2.0) / edited by TB Üstün, N Kostanjsek, S Chatterji, J Rehm.

1.Disability evaluation. 2.Health status. 3.Human development. 4.Classification. 5.Manuals. I.World Health Organization.

ISBN 978 92 4 154759 8 (NLM classification: W 15)

Printed in Malta

Technical editing: Hilary Cadman, Biotext, Canberra, Australia

Contents

Preface

The World Health Organization Disability Assessment Schedule (WHODAS 2.0) is a generic assessment instrument developed by WHO to provide a standardized method for measuring health and disability across cultures. It was developed from a comprehensive set of International Classification of Functioning, Disability and Health (ICF) items that are sufficiently reliable and sensitive to measure the difference made by a given intervention. This is achieved by assessing the same individual before and after the intervention. A series of systematic field studies was used to determine the schedule's cross-cultural applicability, reliability and validity, as well as its utility in health services research. WHODAS 2.0 was found to be useful for assessing health and disability levels in the general population through surveys and for measuring the clinical effectiveness and productivity gains from interventions.

This manual summarizes the methodology used to develop WHODAS 2.0 and the findings obtained when the schedule was applied to certain areas of general health, including mental and neurological disorders. The manual will be useful to any researcher or clinician wishing to use WHODAS 2.0 in their practice. It includes the seven versions of WHODAS 2.0, which differ in length and intended mode of administration. It also provides general population norms; these allow WHODAS 2.0 values for certain subpopulations to be compared with those for the general population.

The manual is aimed at public health professionals, doctors, other health professionals (e.g. rehabilitation professionals, physical therapists and occupational therapists), health-policy planners, social scientists and other individuals involved in studies on disability and health. It may be of particular interest to general health workers, but also to psychiatrists, psychologists, neurologists and addiction health workers, because it places mental health and addiction problems on an equal basis with other areas of general health.

The development of WHODAS 2.0 would not have been possible without the extensive support of many people from different parts of the world, who devoted a great deal of time and energy to the project, and organized resources within an international network. Here, we acknowledge the leading centres, organizations and individuals, and would like to also thank the many other individuals who assisted in different aspects of this large project, which spanned more than 10 years. Further information on the project team is available on the WHODAS 2.0 web site.[1]

WHODAS 2.0 collaborative investigators

The main collaborative investigators, listed by country, were as follows:

Gavin Andrews (Australia), Thomas Kugener (Austria), Kruy Kim Hourn (Cambodia), Yao Guizhong (China), Jesús Saiz (Cuba), Venos Malvreas (Greece), R Srinivasan Murty (India, Bangalore), R Thara (India, Chennai), Hemraj Pal (India, Delhi), Ugo Nocentini and Matilde Leonardi (Italy), Miyako Tazaki (Japan), Elia Karam (Lebanon), Charles Pull (Luxembourg), Hans Wyirand Hoek (The Netherlands), AO Odejide (Nigeria), José Luis Segura Garcia (Peru), Radu Vrasti (Romania), José Luis Vásquez Barquero (Spain), Adel Chaker (Tunisia), Berna Ulug (Turkey), Nick Glozier (United Kingdom), Michael von Korff, Katherine McGonagle and Patrick Doyle (United States of America).

Task Force on Assessment Instruments

The task force included Elizabeth Badley, Cille Kennedy, Ronald Kessler, Michael von Korff, Martin Prince, Karen Ritchie, Ritu Sadana, Gregory Simon, Robert Trotter and Durk Wiersma.

---

[1] http://www.who.int/whodas

WHO/National Institutes for Health Joint Project on Assessment and Classification of Disability

The main people involved in the WHO/National Institutes of Health (NIH) Joint Project on Assessment and Classification of Disability, listed by institution, were as follows: Darrel Regier, Cille Kennedy, Grayson Norquist and Kathy Magruder (National Institute of Mental Health, NIMH); Robert Battjes and Bob Fletcher (National Institute on Drug Abuse, NIDA); and Bridget Grant (National Institute on Alcohol Abuse and Alcoholism, NIAAA).

In addition to the editors, several WHO staff and consultants were part of the WHO/NIH Joint Project; notably, Shekhar Saxena and Joanne Epping-Jordan played key roles. Moreover, we gratefully acknowledge the editorial assistance received from Jayne Lux, Cille Kennedy, Sarah Perini, Rueya Kocalevent and Dan Chisholm, as well as statistical assistance from Ulrich Frick and Luis Prieto.

TB Üstün, N Kostanjsek, S Chatterji, J Rehm

Editors

Abbreviations and acronyms

BAI	Barthel's Index of Activities of Daily Living
CAR	cross-cultural applicability research
CIDI	composite international diagnostic interview
FIM	functional independence measure
GP	general practitioner
ICC	intra-class correlation coefficient
ICF	International Classification of Functioning, Disability and Health
ICF-CY	International Classification of Functioning, Disability and Health Children and Youth version
ICIDH	International Classification of Impairments, Disabilities, and Handicaps
LHS	London Handicap Scale
PCM	partial credit model
SCAN	Schedules for Clinical Assessment in Neuropsychiatry
SF-12	Medical Outcomes Study 12-Item Short-Form Health Survey
SF-36	Medical Outcomes Study 36-Item Short-Form Health Survey
WHO	World Health Organization
WHODAS 2.0	WHO Disability Assessment Schedule
WHOQOL	WHO Quality of Life
WHOQOL-BREF	WHO Quality of Life Brief Scale
WHS	World Health Survey
WMHS	World Mental Health Survey

Part I
Background

1   Introduction

1.1   Why is disability assessment important?

Knowing what disease a patient has requires application of the fine art and science of diagnosis. This knowledge helps to guide treatment interventions and management strategies; it can also help to predict outcome and prognosis to a certain extent. However, although diagnosis is valuable, on its own, it is not sufficient for understanding the full picture and the lived experience of a patient; the adage "there are no diseases, but patients" applies.

Just as important as the disease label itself is whether a person can work and carry out the routine activities necessary to fulfil his or her roles at home, work, school or in other social areas. Summed up by the phrase "what people cannot do when they are ill", this aspect differs greatly, independently of the disease concerned. Information on functioning (i.e. an objective performance in a given life domain) and disability is taken into account by professionals in clinical and social services; however, proper measurement of functioning and disability has long suffered from a lack of consistent definitions and tools. Defining death and disease is easy, but defining disability is difficult, as is measuring it.

Disability is a major health issue. When global assessments are made for burden of disease, more than half of the burden of premature mortality is due to overall disability (1). People generally seek health services because a disease makes it difficult for them to do what they used to do beforehand (i.e. because they are disabled) rather than because they have a disease. Health-care providers consider a case to be clinically significant when it limits a person's daily activities, and they use disability information as the basis of their evaluation and planning.

For public health purposes, disability has become as important as mortality. Although health-care advances have reduced mortality, the associated increase in longevity has led to a corresponding increase in chronic diseases that need to be managed lifelong, and special needs are emerging for the care of aged populations. Public health has to move beyond mortality and take into account disability, to set priorities, measure outcomes and evaluate the effectiveness and performance of health systems. Box 1.1 summarizes the importance of disability assessment.

1.2   Why develop a method to assess disability?

It is difficult to define and measure disability, because disability is related to many life areas, and involves interactions between the person and his or her environment. The World Health Organization (WHO) Project on Assessment and Classification of Human Functioning, Disability and Health brought together representatives of more than 100 countries, researchers and consumers in an international collaboration, to produce the International Classification of Functioning, Disability and Health (ICF) as a consensus framework (2).

The ICF takes each function of an individual – at body, person or society level – and provides a definition for its operational assessment, and defines disability as "a decrement in each functioning domain" (2). However, the ICF is impractical for assessing and measuring disability in daily practice; therefore, WHO developed the WHO Disability Assessment Schedule (WHODAS 2.0) to address this need, and provide a standardized way to measure health and disability across cultures.

Box 1.1 summarizes the reasons for learning and using a disability measure.

Box 1.1 Why learn and use a disability measure?

Diagnosis and assessment of disability is valuable because it can predict the factors that medical diagnosis (assigning a disease label) alone fails to predict; these include:

- service needs – What are the patient's needs?
- level of care – Should the patient be in primary care, specialty care, rehabilitation or another setting?
- outcome of the condition – What will the prognosis be?
- length of hospitalization – How long will the patient stay as an inpatient?
- receipt of disability benefits – Will the patient receive any pension?
- work performance – Will the patient return to work and perform as before?
- social integration – Will the patient return to the community and perform as before?

Disability assessment is thus useful for health care and policy decisions, in terms of:

- identifying needs
- matching treatments and interventions
- measuring outcomes and effectiveness
- setting priorities
- allocating resources.

1.3   What is WHODAS 2.0?

WHODAS 2.0 is a practical, generic assessment instrument that can measure health and disability at population level or in clinical practice. WHODAS 2.0 captures the level of functioning in six domains of life (3):

- Domain 1: Cognition – understanding and communicating
- Domain 2: Mobility – moving and getting around
- Domain 3: Self-care – attending to one's hygiene, dressing, eating and staying alone
- Domain 4: Getting along – interacting with other people
- Domain 5: Life activities – domestic responsibilities, leisure, work and school
- Domain 6: Participation – joining in community activities, participating in society.

The six domains – discussed in detail in Chapter 2 – were selected after a careful review of existing research and survey instruments, and a cross-cultural applicability study.

For all six domains, WHODAS 2.0 provides a profile and a summary measure of functioning and disability that is reliable and applicable across cultures, in all adult populations.

WHODAS 2.0 provides a common metric of the impact of any health condition in terms of functioning. Being a generic measure, the instrument does not target a specific disease – it can thus be used to compare disability due to different diseases. WHODAS 2.0 also makes it possible to design and monitor the impact of health and health-related interventions. The instrument has proven useful for assessing health and disability levels in the general population and in specific groups (e.g. people with a range of different mental and physical conditions). Furthermore, WHODAS 2.0 makes it easier to design health and health-related interventions, and to monitor their impact.

As explained above, WHODAS 2.0 is grounded in the conceptual framework of the ICF. All domains were developed from a comprehensive set of ICF items and map directly onto ICF's "Activity and participation" component (2). As in the ICF, WHODAS 2.0 places health and disability on a continuum, with disability defined as "a decrement in each functioning domain". In addition, WHODAS 2.0, like the ICF, is etiologically neutral; that is, it is independent of the background disease or previous health conditions. This feature makes it possible to focus directly on functioning and disability, and allows the assessment of functioning separately from the disease conditions.

There are several different versions of WHODAS 2.0, which differ in length and intended mode of administration (see Section 2.4 for details). The full version has 36 questions and the short version 12 questions; these questions relate to functioning difficulties experienced by the respondent in the six domains of life during the previous 30 days. The different versions – which are given in Part 3 – can be administered by a lay interviewer, by the person themselves or by a proxy (i.e. family, friend or carer). The 12-item version explains 81% of the variance of the more detailed 36-item version. For both versions, general population norms are available.

1.4   Why use WHODAS 2.0?

There are numerous published measures of disability; these are also known as health status measures or functioning measures. Some of the most widely used measures are summarized in Table 1.1, (pp.6,7). Aspects that make WHODAS 2.0 particularly useful are its sound theoretical underpinnings, good psychometric properties, numerous applications in different groups and settings, and ease of use. This section summarizes the main benefits of WHODAS 2.0.

Direct link to the International Classification of Functioning, Disability and Health

A unique feature of WHODAS 2.0, which distinguishes it from other disability measures, is its direct link to the ICF (2). Although other generic instruments for assessing health status can also be mapped to ICF, they do not clearly distinguish between measurement of symptoms, disability and subjective appraisal. WHODAS 2.0 is unique in that it covers ICF domains fully and applies to all diseases, including physical, mental and substance-use disorders. It also assesses disability in a culturally sensitive way across a standard rating scale. This is discussed in detail in Chapter 2.

Table 1.1 Generic health status and disability assessment instruments

Measure and key references	Background	For use with	Health concepts (domains) measured	No. of items	Administered by	Time to complete (minutes)
WHODAS 2.0 (3–5)	Developed by WHO and based on the ICF. Designed to assess the activity limitations and participation restrictions experienced by an individual, irrespective of medical diagnosis.	Clinical, community and general populations	Cognition Mobility Self-care Getting along Life activities Participation	36	Self or interview	5–10 20
LHS (6)	Based on the descriptive framework of handicap developed by WHO in the ICIDH.	Clinical population only	Mobility Orientation Occupation Physical independence Social integration Economic self-sufficiency	6	Self	5
SF-36 (7–9)	Developed for the Medical Outcomes Study, a study investigating the influence of characteristics of providers, patients and health systems on outcomes of care	Clinical, community and general populations	Physical functioning Role limitations due to physical problems Bodily pain General health perceptions Vitality Social functioning Role limitations due to emotional problems Mental health Health transition	36	Self or interview	10 10
NHP (10,11)	Developed for use in epidemiological studies of health and disease. Designed to reflect the lay perception of health status, rather than the professional definition of health.	Clinical, community and general populations	Energy level Emotional reactions Physical mobility Pain Social isolation Sleep	Part 1: Health problems (38 items) Part 2: Life areas affected (7 items)	Self	5–10

Measure and key references	Background	For use with	Health concepts (domains) measured	No. of items	Administered by	Time to complete (minutes)
FIM (12)	Developed by a task force sponsored by the AAPM&R and the ACRM. Designed to assess the amount of assistance required by a person with a disability to perform basic life activities.	Clinical population only	Self-care Sphincter control Transfers Locomotion Communication Social cognition	18	Interview (by physician, nurse or therapist)	30
BAI (13,14)	Developed in 1955 to assess and monitor mobility and self-care activities of daily living.	Clinical population only	Bowel status Bladder status Grooming Toilet use[a] Feeding Transfers[a] Mobility[a] Dressing Stairs[a] Bathing[a]	5–10	Interview (by therapist or other observer)	2–5

AAPM&R, American Academy of Physical Medicine and Rehabilitation; ACRM, American Congress of Rehabilitation Medicine; BAI, Barthel's Index of Activities of Daily Living; FIM, Functional Independence Measure; ICF, International Classification of Functioning, Disability and Health; ICIDH, International Classification of Impairments, Disabilities, and Handicaps; LHS, London Handicap Scale; NHP, Nottingham Health Profile; SF-36, Medical Outcomes Study 36-Item Short-Form Health Survey; WHODAS 2.0, WHO Disability Assessment Schedule 2.0
[a] Items included in 5-item version.

Cross-cultural comparability

Unlike other disability measures, WHODAS 2.0 was developed on the basis of an extensive cross-cultural study, spanning 19 countries across the world. The items included in WHODAS 2.0 were selected only after exploring the nature and practice of health status assessment in different cultures. This was achieved using a linguistic analysis of health-related terminology, key informant interviews and focus groups, as well as qualitative methods (e.g. pile sorting and concept mapping[1]) (3). Once developed, WHODAS 2.0 was tested in a variety of different cultural settings and health populations, and was found to be sensitive to change, regardless of the sociodemographic profile of the study group.

Psychometric properties

WHODAS 2.0 has excellent psychometric properties. Test–retest studies of the 36-item scale in countries across the world found it to be highly reliable. All items were selected on the basis of item–response theory (i.e. the application of mathematical models to data gathered from questionnaires and tests). The instrument as a whole showed a robust factor structure (see Section 3.2) that remained constant across cultures and different types of patient populations. The validation studies also showed that WHODAS 2.0 compared well with other measures of disability or health status, and with clinician and proxy ratings (15,16).

Ease of use and availability

WHODAS 2.0 can be self-administered in around 5 minutes, and administered through an interview in 20 minutes. The instrument is easy to score and interpret, is in the public domain, and is available in more than 30 languages.

1.5 Purpose and structure of the manual

1.5.1 Purpose

This manual is aimed at health professionals (e.g. in the areas of public health, rehabilitation, physical therapy and occupational therapy), health-policy planners, social scientists and other individuals involved in studies on disability and health. It will provide users with:

- a new appreciation of health status and disability assessment in the light of the framework and classification provided by the ICF;
- a detailed overview of the development, key features and application of WHODAS 2.0; and
- a comprehensive guide to administering the various versions of WHODAS 2.0 correctly and effectively.

---

[1] "Pile sorting" refers to a research technique in which individuals list topics relevant to a particular subject, then group listed topics into related piles. "Concept mapping" refers to the creation of a concept map, which is used to explore knowledge or to gather and share information. The map consists of nodes or cells, each of which contains a concept, item or question. The nodes are linked by arrows that are labelled to explain how they relate to one another.

1.5.2 Structure

This manual is organized into three parts, covering background information (Part 1), administration and scoring of the instrument (Part 2) and the different versions of WHODAS 2.0 (Part 3).

The contents of Chapters 2–4, which make up the remainder of Part 1, are as follows:

*   *Chapter 2* discusses the development of WHODAS 2.0 – the rationale and conceptual background for its development, and the method and stages of the development process. This chapter also introduces the different versions of WHODAS 2.0, and the schedule's methods, sources and major findings. It covers the technical basis and implications of incorporating disability into health assessments, and provides more detail on the links between the ICF and WHODAS 2.0.
*   *Chapter 3* focuses on the psychometric properties of WHODAS 2.0. It discusses the instrument's reliability and consistency, the factor structure, sensitivity to change, item–response characteristics, validity and general population properties.
*   *Chapter 4* outlines the uses of WHODAS 2.0 at population and clinical levels. It looks at how the instrument can be used in population surveys and registers, and for monitoring outcomes for individual patients in clinical practice and clinical trials of treatment effects.

Part 2 has a practical focus. It contains six chapters:

*   *Chapter 5* presents generic information and instructions for the different modes of administering WHODAS 2.0, general guidelines for the application of the instrument and guidance on developing versions in different languages.
*   *Chapter 6* covers the scoring of WHODAS 2.0. It includes information on sample characteristics, computing items, domain and summary scores, population norms and handling of missing data.
*   *Chapters 7–10* provide question-by-question specifications for all six domains, detailed guidelines for using the various WHODAS 2.0 versions, material for self-testing and a sample training curriculum.

At the end of Part 2, there is a glossary and a list of references.

As mentioned above, Part 3 of this manual provides the seven different versions of WHODAS 2.0.

2 WHODAS 2.0 development

This chapter discusses the development of WHODAS 2.0 – the rationale and conceptual background for its development, and the method and stages of the development process. It also introduces the different versions of WHODAS 2.0 and the schedule's methods, sources and major findings. The chapter covers the technical basis and implications of incorporating disability into health assessments, and expands on the information given in Chapter 1 about the links between the ICF and WHODAS 2.0.

2.1 Rationale and conceptual background for the development of WHODAS 2.0

The original Disability Assessment Schedule WHO/DAS – published by WHO in 1988 – was an instrument developed to assess functioning, mainly in psychiatric inpatients (17–20). Since then, the instrument has undergone considerable revision by the WHO Collaborating Centre at Groningen in The Netherlands, and been published as the "Groningen Social Disabilities Schedule" (GSDS) (21,22).

WHODAS 2.0 is an altogether different instrument that has been developed specifically to reflect the ICF. WHO developed the ICF as both a health classification and a model of the complete experience of disability. The disability statistics in the ICF provide measures for assessing the disability burden of all health conditions, both physical and mental, whatever their cause.

Structurally, the ICF is based on three levels of functioning, with parallel levels of disability, as shown in Table 2.1.

Table 2.1 Levels of functioning and disability used in the International Classification of Functioning, Disability and Health (ICF)(2)

Level of functioning	Parallel level of disability
Body functions and structures	Impairments
Activities	Activity limitations
Participation	Participation restrictions

Human functioning is understood as a continuum of health states, and everyone exhibits some degree of functioning in each domain, at the level of the body, the person and society.

The ICF conceptualizes disability as a health experience that occurs in a context, rather than as a problem that resides solely in the individual. According to the biopsychosocial model embedded in the ICF, disability and functioning are outcomes of interactions between health conditions (diseases, disorders and injuries) and contextual factors. The model recognizes that disability is multidimensional and is the product of an interaction between attributes of an individual and features of the person's physical, social and attitudinal environment. It broadens the perspective of disability and allows for the examination of medical, individual, social and environmental influences on functioning and disability.

The authors of this manual strongly recommend that users of WHODAS 2.0 read the introduction to the ICF and the accompanying educational materials, which are available on the WHO web site.[1]

WHODAS 2.0 aims to reflect the key features of the ICF. It has been designed to assess the limitations on activity and restrictions on participation experienced by an individual, irrespective of medical diagnosis.

WHODAS 2.0 was developed through collaborations between WHO and the following organizations from the United States of America – the National Institutes of Health (NIH), the National Institute of Mental Health (NIMH), the National Institute on Alcohol Abuse and Alcoholism (NIAAA) and the National In-

---

[1] http://www.who.int/classifications/icf

stitute on Drug Abuse (NIDA). The project is referred to as the WHO/NIH Joint Project on Assessment and Classification of Disability.

2.2 Relation with WHO Quality of Life instrument

WHO has also developed the Quality of Life (WHOQOL[1]) instrument, which assesses subjective well-being in different areas of life (23). Conceptually, the constructs of quality of life and functioning are often seen as interchangeable. Although these constructs are indeed interrelated, WHODAS 2.0 measures functioning (i.e. an objective performance in a given life domain), while WHOQOL measures subjective well-being (i.e. a feeling of satisfaction about one's performance in a given life domain). Ideally, the same life domains should be used in both instruments. Whereas WHODAS 2.0 asks what a person "does" in a particular domain, WHOQOL asks what the person "feels" in that domain.

2.3 Process of development of WHODAS 2.0

The method used to develop WHODAS 2.0 had several unique features; these were:

- a collaborative international approach, with the aim of developing a single generic instrument for assessing health status and disability in different settings (discussed in detail below);
- a unique set of cross-cultural applicability study protocols, to ensure that WHODAS 2.0 would have a high degree of functional and metric equivalence across different cultures and settings; and
- a connection with the revision of the ICF, to allow the new instrument to be directly linked to the ICF.

Collaborative approach

Several culturally diverse centres were involved in operationalizing the instrument's six domains, writing and selecting questions, deriving response scales and carrying out pilot testing. Thus, issues such as standardization, equivalence between settings and translation were at the forefront of the development process. To ensure that the collaboration was genuinely international, field centres were selected based on differences in settings, level of industrialization, available health services and other markers relevant to the measurement of health and disability (e.g. role of the family, perception of time, and perception of self and dominant religion).

The extensive and rigorous international research involved in developing WHODAS 2.0 included:

- a critical review of the literature on conceptualization and measurement of functioning and disability, and of related instruments (24,25);
- a systematic cross-cultural applicability study (3); and
- a series of empirical field studies to develop and refine the instrument.

These steps are discussed below.

Review of existing instruments

In preparation for the development of WHODAS 2.0, WHO assembled a Task Force on Assessment Instruments, comprising international experts, to review existing instruments. The task force chose a broad range of instruments, including various measures of disability, handicap, quality of life and other health status (e.g. activities of daily living, instrumental activities of daily living, global or specific measures, subjective well-being and quality of life). The 300 or so instruments reviewed reflected considerable diversity in terms of theoretical framework, terminology, constructs measured, assessment strategy, level of skills assessed, assessment goals and focus of valuation. Despite this diversity, it was possible to refine a pool of "items" (i.e. core domains of functioning and disability), and link them to the ICF.

Information about the instruments was compiled into a database showing the common pool of items, and their origin and known psychometric properties. Over two years, the task force reviewed the data and the pool of items, using the ICF as the common framework. Undertaking the review enabled the con-

---

[1]   http://www.who.int/whoqol

struction of WHODAS 2.0 to benefit from the knowledge base of all existing assessment instruments; it also meant that the new instrument was congruent with the revised ICF.

After careful deliberation and initial pilot tests (see below), the task force grouped the items into the following six domains:

- *Domain 1: Cognition* – Assesses communication and thinking activities; specific areas assessed include concentrating, remembering, problem solving, learning and communicating.

- *Domain 2: Mobility* – Assesses activities such as standing, moving around inside the home, getting out of the home and walking a long distance.

- *Domain 3: Self-care* – Assesses hygiene, dressing, eating and staying alone.

- *Domain 4: Getting along* – Assesses interactions with other people and difficulties that might be encountered with this life domain due to a health condition; in this context, "other people" includes those known intimately or well (e.g. spouse or partner, family members or close friends) and those not known well (e.g. strangers).

- *Domain 5: Life activities* – Assesses difficulty with day-to-day activities (i.e. those that people do on most days, including those associated with domestic responsibilities, leisure, work and school).

- *Domain 6: Participation* – Assesses social dimensions, such as community activities; barriers and hindrances in the world around the respondent; and problems with other issues, such as maintaining personal dignity. The questions do not necessarily and solely refer to the ICF participation component as such, but also include various contextual (personal and environmental) factors affected by the health condition of the respondent.

Cross-cultural applicability study

To ensure that WHODAS 2.0 is cross-culturally meaningful and valid, a systematic research study was undertaken. The cross-cultural applicability research (CAR) study used various qualitative methods to explore the nature and practice of health status assessment in different cultures (*3*). The study included linguistic analysis of health-related terminology, key informant interviews, focus groups and quasi-quantitative methods such as pile sorting and concept mapping (carried out in tandem). Information was gathered on the conceptualization of disability and on important areas of day-to-day functioning.

The study provided rich insights into the constructs that were likely to be universally applicable, possible anchors for the domain scales and thresholds for the assessment instrument, and phraseology and dimensions that could be used in the assessment instruments. It also highlighted areas that might require more careful probing and attention in order to construct reliable and valid instruments, as well as issues related to parity between physical and mental conditions that needed to be addressed. The study led to the production of a version of WHODAS 2.0 with 96 items grouped into 6 domains, to be used in formative field studies; the studies were designed to reduce the number of items and increase reliability.

Reliability and validity field studies

The psychometric properties of WHODAS 2.0 were subject to two waves of international testing, using a multicentre design with identical protocols, as summarized in Box 2.1 and 2.2. Study sites were chosen for their geographic representation of different WHO regions (taking into account cultural and linguistic variation) and their suitability for reaching different populations and conducting research. In each phase, the general study design required equal numbers of subjects at each site to be drawn from four different groups:

- general population;
- populations with physical problems;
- populations with mental or emotional problems; and
- populations with problems related to alcohol and drug use.

Each site recruited subjects 18 years or older, with gender evenly distributed. Each subject was given a description of the study and informed consent was obtained as set forth by the ethical standards of WHO.

In Domain 5 – life activities – samples included people who were employed, self-employed, retired or not working. Therefore, all results were grouped into two main categories: work sample (i.e. people who reported gainful employment) and overall sample. WHODAS 2.0 scores for Domain 5 are therefore calculated separately for the sections that cover the work sample.

Box 2.1 WHODAS 2.0 field studies: Item reduction and feasibility

Study sites

Studies were undertaken at the 21 sites listed below.

Site	n	Site	n
Austria (Innsbruck)	50	Netherlands (The Hague)	47
Cambodia (Phnom Penh)	50	Nigeria (Ibadan)	50
China (Beijing)	50	Peru (Lima)	59
Cuba (Havana)	50	Romania (Timisoara)	50
Greece (Athens)	48	Spain (Santander)	54
India 1 (Bangalore)	283	Tunisia (Tunis)	50
India 2 (Delhi)	154	Turkey (Ankara)	49
Italy (Rome)	20	United Kingdom (London)	35
Japan	50	United States of America 1 (Michigan)	152
Lebanon	37	United States of America 2 (Seattle)	43
Luxembourg (Luxembourg)	50		

Characteristics of sample

	n	%
Origin:		
General population	262	18.3
Physical problems	418	29.3
Mental or emotional problems	394	27.6
Alcohol-related problems	195	13.6
Drug-use-related problems	162	11.3
Sex:		
Female	651	45.5
Male	780	54.5
Age:		
Under 55 years	1078	75.3
55 years and above	353	24.7

Methodological Study 1 on different ways to ascertain duration of disability (total *n* = 651):

Study sites

Studies were undertaken at the seven sites listed below.

Site	n	Site	n
Cambodia (Phnom Penh)	100	Lebanon (Beirut)	50
Germany (Hamburg)	69	Romania (Timisoara)	101
India (Bangalore)	138	Tunisia (Tunis)	100
India (Delhi)	93		

Methodological Study 2 on comparison standard (explicit versus implicit) (total *n* = 396):

Studies were undertaken at one site, in India (Bangalore).

Box 2.2 WHODAS 2.0 field studies: Reliability and validity

Study sites

Studies were undertaken at the 16 sites listed below.

Site	n	Site	n
Austria (Innsbruck)	100	Luxembourg (Luxembourg)	98
Cambodia (Phnom Penh)	98	Netherlands (The Hague)	50
China (Beijing)	100	Nigeria (Ibadan)	140
Greece (Athens)	96	Romania (Timisoara)	108
India 1 (Bangalore)	100	Russian Federation (Moscow)	105
India 2 (Chennai)	100	Spain (Santander)	99
India 2 (Delhi)	95	Tunisia (Tunis)	123
Italy (Rome)	96	United States of America (multiple)	57

Characteristics of sample

	n	%
Origin:		
General population	366	23.4
Physical problems	405	25.9
Mental or emotional problems	402	25.7
Alcohol-related problems	225	14.4
Drug-use-related problems	167	10.7
Sex:		
Female	641	41.0
Male	924	59.0
Age:		
Under 55 years	1304	83.3
55 years and above	261	16.7

Wave 1 studies (see Box 2.1) first used the 96-item version of WHODAS 2.0 to obtain empirical feedback. This feedback could be used to determine which items were redundant, the performance of the short version, and the applicability of the rating scales and the timeframe. Eight steps were involved in these studies:

1. Complete language translation and back-translation of the instrument and supporting material, with linguistic analysis of difficulties encountered.

2. Application of the WHODAS 2.0 interview.

3. Collection of additional data on the feasibility of the interview and on diagnosis.

4. Cognitive debriefing protocol and qualitative surveys with subjects, interviewers and other experts.

5. Focus groups on WHODAS 2.0.

6. Concurrent application of Medical Outcomes Study 12-Item Short-Form Health Survey (SF-12), and the 36-item version (SF-36) (*7,26*), and the London Handicap Scale (LHS) (*6*).

7. Concurrent application of WHOQOL(*23*) or the WHOQOL Brief Scale (WHOQOL–BREF) (*27*).

8. Optional use of ICF checklist (*28*).

Data analysis of Wave 1 studies focused on reducing the number of items from 96 to a more reasonable number, and examining the psychometric properties of questions and the factor structures that would allow the instrument to be shortened but would maintain the six domains.

The following criteria were used to select the final items of WHODAS 2.0:

- cultural acceptance, which was assessed based on the qualitative components of field trials (expert opinion, cognitive debriefing, interviewer feedback) and on a quantitative analysis of missing values (e.g. certain items having more than 10% missing values in certain cultures) (29);

- factor loading, which needed to be higher than 0.6 in the domains where the item was placed (4);

- minimal cross-loading of items (i.e. loading in more than one domain);

- high discriminatory power at all levels, assessed using models derived from item-response theory (non-parametric approaches such as Mokken (30) and parametric approaches such as the Birnbaum model (31)); and

- minimal redundancy (e.g. eliminating of one of two related items, such as "standing for a short period" and "standing for a long period").

On the basis of classical test theory and item-response theory analysis, the 96-item version was reduced to 34 items (4). Two further items were then added, based on input received from interviewers in the field and from the expert opinion survey – one of the additional items related to limitations in sexual activities and one to the impact of the health condition on the family.

Wave 2 studies involved testing the revised version's psychometric properties across different sites and populations, as summarized in Box 2.2 (4,15). The psychometric properties of the WHODAS 2.0 36-item version are summarized in Chapter 3.

2.4   Final structure of WHODAS 2.0

Three versions of WHODAS 2.0 were developed – a 36-item, 12-item and 12+24-item version, each of which is discussed below. All the versions query functioning difficulties in the six selected domains (listed in Section 2.3, above) during the 30 days preceding the interview.

Depending on the information needed, the study design and the time constraints, the user can choose between three versions of WHODAS 2.0.

36-item version

Of the three versions, the 36-item version of WHODAS 2.0 is the most detailed. It allows users to generate scores for the six domains of functioning and to calculate an overall functioning score.

For each item that is positively endorsed, a follow-up question asks about the number of days (in the past 30 days) on which the respondent has experienced the particular difficulty. The 36-item version is available in three different forms – interviewer-administered, self-administered and proxy-administered.

The average interview time for the interviewer-administered 36-item version is 20 minutes.

12-item version

The 12-item version of WHODAS 2.0 is useful for brief assessments of overall functioning in surveys or health-outcome studies in situations where time constraints do not allow for application of the longer version. The 12-item version explains 81% of the variance of the 36-item version. As with the 36-item version, the 12-item version is available in three different forms – interviewer-administered, self-administered and proxy-administered.

The average interview time for the interviewer-administered 12-item version is five minutes.

12+24-item version

The 12+24-item version of WHODAS 2.0 is a simple hybrid of the 12-item and 36-item versions. It uses 12 items to screen for problematic domains of functioning. Based on positive responses to the initial 12 items, respondents may be given up to 24 additional questions. Thus, this is a simple, adaptive test that attempts to capture 36 items fully, while avoiding negative responses. The 12+24-item version can only be administered by interview or computer-adaptive testing (CAT).

For each item that is positively endorsed, a follow-up question asks about the number of days (in the past 30 days) the respondent has experienced this difficulty. The average interview time for the 12+24-item version is 20 minutes.

3 Psychometric properties of WHODAS 2.0

This chapter reports on the psychometric properties of WHODAS 2.0. It discusses the extensive field tests conducted in countries across the world, which revealed that WHODAS 2.0 has good reliability and item-response characteristics, and a sturdy factor structure that remains consistent across cultures and different types of patient populations. This chapter also discusses the validity studies, which showed that the results obtained with WHODAS 2.0 are consistent with those from other measures of disability or health status, or with clinician and proxy ratings.

3.1 Test–retest reliability and internal consistency

As explained in Chapter 2, test–retest reliability and internal consistency of WHODAS 2.0 were determined during the Wave 2 studies. A standard test–retest design was used, with the second application session occurring within seven days of the first interview (mean interval, 2.4 ± 1.6 days) to maximize the overlap in the timeframes of reference of the two interviews. First and second interviews were completed by different interviewers.

Results of the reliability analysis are shown in Figure 3.1 as a summary for item, domain and full instrument (overall) levels. Test–retest reliability had an intra-class coefficient of 0.69–0.89 at item level; 0.93–0.96 at domain level; and 0.98 at overall level.

Figure 3.1   WHODAS 2.0 reliability: test–retest summary[a]

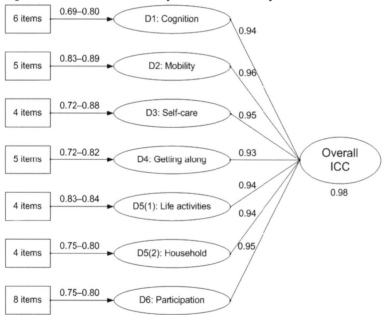

D, domain; ICC, intra-class coefficient

[a] Wave 2 (n_{total} = 1565; n_s for ICC depend on domain; for example, on how many subjects responded to all items at both time points: D1, 1448; D2, 1529; D3, 1430; D4, 1222; D5(1), 1399; D5(2) – only with remunerated work, 808; D6, 1431.

Internal consistencies at the domain and summary levels, based on responses at first interview (time 1), were examined using item–total correlations and Cronbach's alphas[1] (which measure how well a set of variables or items measures a single, unidimensional latent construct). In general, these values ranged from "acceptable" to "very good". Ranges for item–total values for the overall sample were as shown in Table 3.1.

---

[1]   Cronbach's alpha is a measure of of well a set of variables or items measures a single, unidimensional latent construct.

Table 3.1 Ranges for item–total values for the overall sample

Domain	Range
1	0.59–0.70
2	0.74–0.79
3	0.47–0.73
4	0.52–0.76
5	0.88–0.94
6	0.54–0.74

Cronbach's alpha levels were generally very high, as can be seen in Table 3.2.

Table 3.2 Cronbach's alpha values for WHODAS 2.0 domain[a] and total scores, of the overall sample and by subgroup

	Domain							
	1	2	3	4	5(1)	5(2)	6	Total score
n	1444	1524	1425	1217	1396	807	1428	578
Overall Cronbach's alpha *n* = 1565	0.94	0.96	0.95	0.94	0.94	0.94	0.95	0.98
Population group								
General	0.93	0.96	0.94	0.93	0.91	0.95	0.93	0.97
Drug	0.91	0.94	0.92	0.88	0.92	0.89	0.94	0.98
Alcohol	0.93	0.91	0.87	0.94	0.93	0.90	0.93	0.98
Mental	0.94	0.93	0.92	0.94	0.92	0.94	0.93	0.98
Physical	0.92	0.96	0.96	0.92	0.95	0.94	0.94	0.97
Gender								
Female	0.95	0.96	0.95	0.96	0.94	0.96	0.97	0.99
Male	0.92	0.96	0.95	0.91	0.94	0.93	0.94	0.98
Age								
< 55 years	0.94	0.96	0.95	0.94	0.94	0.94	0.96	0.98
≥55 years	0.90	0.95	0.94	0.93	0.93	0.99	0.95	0.99

[a] Domains – 1: Cognition; 2: Mobility; 3: Self-care; 4: Getting along; 5(1): Life activities (household); 5(2): Life activities (work); 6: Participation

3.2 Factor structure

Wave 1 factor analysis revealed a two-level hierarchical structure, with one general disability factor feeding into the six domains (see Figure 3.2). Most questions fitted best in their theoretically assigned domains, confirming the unidimensionality of domains; the exception was leisure questions in Domain 5 (life activities), which actually belong in Domain 6.

Variance explained by a first general factor was as follows:

- Domain 1 (cognition) – 47%
- Domain 2 (mobility) – 54%
- Domain 3 (self-care) – 54%
- Domain 4 (getting along) – 62%
- Domain 5 (life activities) – 31%
- Domain 6 (participation) – 51%.

Confirmatory factor analysis showed a rigorous association between the factor structure of the items and the domains, and between the domains and a general disability factor. These results again support the unidimensionality of domains. The factor structure was similar across the different study sites and populations tested. Wave 2 factor analysis essentially replicated these results.

Figure 3.2   WHODAS 2.0 factor structure [a]

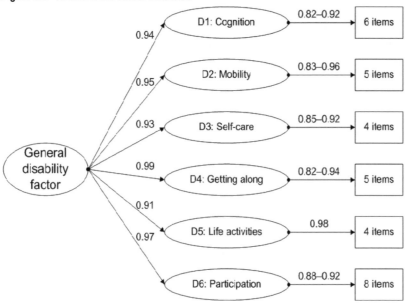

[a] Wave 1 confirmatory factor analysis (*n* = 1050 without the work section)

3.3   Cross-cultural sensitivity to change

WHODAS 2.0 responsiveness studies have been conducted in a variety of health populations and treatment settings throughout the world; results are shown in Figure 3.3. All of the studies followed a common protocol, in which the 36-item, interview version of WHODAS 2.0 was administered on at least two occasions – once on entry to the study and again at follow-up assessment (at least four weeks later). In each of the studies, another disability measure (e.g. LHS or SF-36 – see Table 1.1 in Chapter 1) was also administered at both time points, and disorder severity was assessed based on the clinician's judgement or a standardized measure (e.g. Clinical Global Impression, Hamilton Depression Rating Scale).

Figure 3.3   WHODAS 2.0 percentage reduction at follow-up assessment

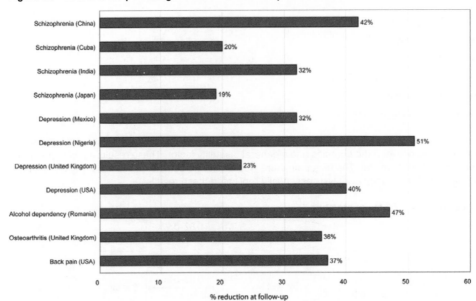

Overall, WHODAS 2.0 was found to be at least as sensitive to change as other measures of social functioning, with study-specific effect sizes ranging from 0.46 for outpatient care of the depressed elderly in the United Kingdom to 1.38 for outpatient care of newly referred schizophrenia cases in China (29). Figure 3.3 also shows the reduction of WHODAS 2.0 scores in each of the studies. A pooled multilevel analysis of subjects across the different studies revealed that summary change scores were unaffected by sociodemographic factors, suggesting that WHODAS 2.0 is applicable across cultures.

3.4   Item-response characteristics

In Wave 2 studies, WHODAS 2.0 items were tested in a dichotomized version – none (rated as "0") versus any limitation (rated as "1", "2", "3", "4") – as well as in their original 5-point Likert-scale version. For dichotomous items, the Rasch model was fitted to both samples and both versions (i.e. including work items versus excluding work items). For polytomous items, the assumption of ordinal item steps was assessed by inspecting the conditional transition probabilities between adjacent categories estimated for a partial credit model (which can be seen as a polytomous extension of a Rasch scale).

The results of the studies indicated that the dichotomous version of WHODAS 2.0 was compatible with Rasch assumptions, and the polytomous version was compatible with the partial credit model, provided that a number of items were recoded (see Chapter 6).

3.5   Validity

Face validity

In terms of face validity – that is, the indicators that show that the instrument measures what it is intended to measure – 64% of the experts agreed that the WHODAS 2.0 content measures disability as defined by the ICF.

Measurement properties of WHODAS 2.0 that emerged across treatment categories showed meaningful scores in expected directions. All treatment groups (drug, alcohol, physical and mental) scored significantly higher (i.e. had greater disability) than the general population group, indicating that WHODAS 2.0 is sensitive to functional problems across a range of underlying diseases and disorders. Within treatment groups, the domain profiles were consistent with what might be expected. For example, the physical group scored significantly worse than all other groups on the domains that emphasize mobility (i.e. mobility [Domain 2] and self-care [Domain 3]), whereas the drug group scored significantly worse than other groups on participation in society (Domain 6). Figure 3.4 shows the domain profiles across subgroups.

Figure 3.4 WHODAS 2.0 domain profile by subgroup

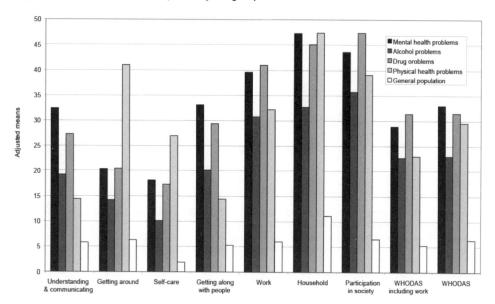

Concurrent validity

In the Wave 2 studies, WHODAS 2.0 was administered simultaneously with other known instruments such as the LHS, the Medical Outcomes Study's 36-Item Health Survey (SF-36), SF-12, the Functional Independence Measure (FIM), WHOQOL-100 and WHOQOL-BREF, in different countries and populations *(15)*. Table 3.3 summarizes these results, showing correlation coefficients with relevant domains from the LHS, FIM and SF. As expected, the highest correlations were found with specific domains measuring similar constructs; in particular, between the FIM and WHODAS 2.0 mobility domains. Other correlations were mostly between 0.45 and 0.65, indicating similarity of constructs between WHODAS 2.0 dimensions and recognized tests, but also that WHODAS 2.0 is measuring something distinct.

Table 3.3 Correlation coefficients between WHODAS 2.0 and related instruments

WHODAS 2.0 domain	SF-36 (n = 608–658)/ SF-12 (n = 93–94) [a,b]	WHOQOL (n = 257–288)	LHS (n = 662–839)	FIM[c] (n = 68–82)
1 – Cognition	−0.19 / −0.10	−0.50	−0.62	−0.53
2 – Getting around	−0.68 / −0.69	−0.50	−0.53	−0.78
3 – Self-care	−0.55 / −0.52	−0.48	−0.58	−0.75
4 – Getting along	−0.21 / −0.21	−0.54	−0.50	−0.34
5(1) – Life activities (household)	−0.54 / −0.46	−0.57	−0.64	−0.60
5(2) – Life activities (work)	−0.59 / −0.64 (n = 372/42)	−0.63 (n = 166)	−0.52 (n = 498)	−0.52 (n = 23)
6 – Participation	−0.55 / −0.43	−0.66	−0.64	−0.62

FIM, Functional Independence Measure; LHS, London Handicap Scale; SF-12, Medical Outcomes Study 12-Item Short-Form Health Survey; SF-36, Medical Outcomes Study 36-Item Short-Form Health Survey; WHOQOL, WHO Quality of Life Project.

[a] Numbers in parentheses are the minimum and maximum number of subjects the correlations are based on. Since the n for "work" has been considerably lower, because this set of questions has only been given to people with remunerated work, these results are given separately.

[b] For correlations with WHODAS 2.0 Domains 1 and 4, the SF mental scores were used; for all other domains, the SF physical scores were used.

[c] For Domain 1, the FIM cognition score was used as basis of the correlation; for Domain 2, FIM mobility was used; for all other domains, the overall FIM score was used.

Construct validity

Construct validity involves explicitly specifying the dimensions of the construct of interest, the area covered by the dimensions (both uniquely and jointly) and the expected relations of the dimensions to each other (both internally and externally). Evidence of construct validity can be seen from the extent to which a new measure correlates with an existing measure of the same construct, and differentiates from a third, distantly related measure.

Construct validity is the degree to which inferences made from a study can be generalized to the underlying concepts (32). In accordance with this definition, WHODAS 2.0 has construct validity. In people who have certain health conditions (e.g. cataract, hip or knee problems, depression, schizophrenia or alcohol problems), WHODAS 2.0 can pick up improvements in functioning following treatment. This feature is also called "sensitivity to change" or "responsiveness of an instrument" (see Section 3.3). In accordance with the health services research studies conducted within the WHODAS 2.0 field trials (29), WHODAS 2.0 was sufficiently sensitive to pick up change in the functioning profiles of the treatment group. This change was statistically significant and comparable to, or better than, other established measures commonly used in the field for similar purposes. Figure 3.5 illustrates the sensitivity to change of WHODAS 2.0 in people who receive treatment for depression.

Figure 3.5   WHODAS 2.0 sensitivity to change (responsiveness) in cases receiving depression treatment (*29*)

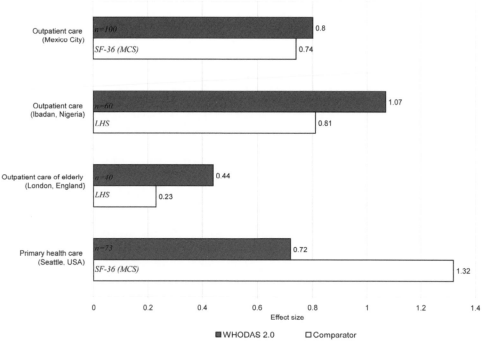

LHS, London Handicap Scale; SF-36, Medical Outcomes Study 36-Item Short-Form Health Survey; MCS, mental component summary
Note: Results are reported as effect size (change in mean/SD1), see Glossary

3.6   WHODAS 2.0 in the general population

Following the demonstration of the reliability and concurrent validity of WHODAS 2.0, a study was launched to test the properties of the instrument in large general population surveys, and to establish the norms for scoring WHODAS 2.0. This study was carried out in China, Colombia, Egypt, Georgia, India, Indonesia, Islamic Republic of Iran, Lebanon, Mexico, Nigeria, Singapore, Slovakia, Syria and Turkey, as a part of the WHO Multi-Country Survey Study on Health and Responsiveness 2000–2001 (MCSS) (*34*). The samples were selected using probabilistic methods, and were nationally or regionally representative. The survey included 21 items from the WHODAS 2.0 36-item version; it measured self-reported health status, and included performance tests for cognition, mobility and vision.

The MCSS demonstrated the feasibility of the use of the WHODAS 2.0 in the general population, and showed that the instrument has the same psychometric properties in different population groups. It also provided the data for the normative scores against which different study populations can now be compared.

Subsequently, based on the results of the MCSS, the same concepts were also applied in the WHO World Health Surveys (WHS) that were carried out in 70 countries. The usefulness of these constructs was once again established (*35*). Since then, the instrument has also been used in a modified form in the WHO World Mental Health Surveys, to measure the impact of mental and physical disorders (*36,37*).

4 Uses of WHODAS 2.0

This chapter outlines the uses of WHODAS 2.0 at population and clinical levels. For example, it looks at how the instrument can be used in population surveys and registers, and for monitoring outcomes for individual patients in clinical practice and clinical trials of treatment effects.

4.1 Applications of WHODAS 2.0

WHODAS 2.0 was conceived as a general health state assessment measure, capable of being used for multiple purposes and in different settings. Table 4.1 contains summaries of WHODAS 2.0 applications in surveys of general and specific populations. Further information on WHODAS 2.0 applications is provided in a user database on the WHODAS 2.0 web site.[1]

Table 4.1 Population survey applications of WHODAS 2.0

Application name	Summary of application
Multi-Country Survey Study on Health and Responsiveness 2000–2001 (MCSS) and World Health Survey (WHS)	**Population characteristics:** Nationally representative face-to-face household surveys. MCSS conducted in 10 countries (n = 130 000), WHS conducted in 70 countries (n = 240 000). **WHODAS 2.0 version used:** MCSS: 12-item version and selected items from 36-item version and level of impairment question module; WHS: adapted 12-item version and impairment question module. **Main findings:** Validation of WHODAS 2.0 population norms; domain specific and overall level of functioning and disability prevalence (*34,35*).
World Mental Health Survey (WMHS)	**Population characteristics:** Nationally representative sample of adult population (n = 12 992). **WHODAS 2.0 version used:** 12-item version. **Main findings:** Assessed the factor structure, internal consistency, and discriminatory validity of the WHODAS 2.0 version used in the European Study of the Epidemiology of Mental Disorders (*38*). Findings from other sub-studies: • Examined and compared the association of mental and physical disorders with multiple domains of functioning. WHODAS 2.0 was used to measure functional status, with the WHO Composite International Diagnostic Interview (CIDI) used as the measure for mental disorders (*39,40*). • Results show a strong impact of mental health state and specific mental and physical disorders on work-role disability and quality of life in six European countries (*41*).
Global Study on Ageing	**Population characteristics:** Longitudinal survey programme with an emphasis on populations aged 50+ years, from nationally representative samples in six countries (China, Ghana, India, Mexico, Russian Federation and South Africa). **WHODAS 2.0 version used:** 12-item version. **Main findings:** Ongoing.
WHO/United Nations Economic and Social Commission for Asia and the Pacific (UNESACAP) project on improving disability statistics	**Population characteristics:** Prototypical sample of general population in five countries (Fiji, India, Indonesia, Mongolia and Philippines). **WHODAS 2.0 version used:** 36-item version and level of impairment question module of the WHS. **Main findings:** WHODAS 2.0 and WHS questions showed good specificity and sensitivity, predictive validity, reliability, translatability and cognitive understanding across cultures. Questions were recommended to be part of a disability questions module for census and surveys (*42*).

---

[1]   http://www.who.int/whodas

Ireland's National Physical and Sensory Disability Database (NPSDD)	**Population characteristics:** National population currently registered in the database (n = 5191). **WHODAS 2.0 version used:** 12-item version. **Main findings:** WHODAS 2.0 is used as part of an indicator set for routine reporting in Ireland's National Physical and Sensory Disability Database. The database provides disability profiles of the registered population across the WHODAS 2.0 domains (*43,44*).
Nicaraguan Survey for People with Disability	**Population characteristics:** National and subnational representative sample. **WHODAS version used:** 36-item version. **Main findings:** Disability prevalence was measured using tools based on WHODAS 2.0. Disability prevalence was higher than previous estimations; other estimations focused on deficiencies. This study showed the usefulness of the ICF and WHODAS 2.0 (*45*).
Perfomance Assessment National Survey (Mexico)	**Population characteristics:** National and subnational representative sample (n = 39 000 households). **WHODAS version used:** 36-item; the survey includes measurements of eight health domains. **Main findings:** Using the WHODAS 2.0 scoring algorithm, prevalence of disability was estimated for national and subnational levels. The results demonstrated the usefulness of an ICF-based measurement approach at population level. In addition, the results were used as inputs to estimate healthy life expectancy at national and subnational levels (*46*).
FIrst National Study on Disability (Chile)	**Population characteristics:** National and subnational representative sample (n = 13 350 households). **WHODAS version used:** 36-item . **Main findings:** Based on WHODAS 2.0, disability prevalence and severity levels were estimated for national and regional levels. The results were useful in understanding the nature and scope of disability in Chile, and have been useful for policy making and resource allocation (*47*).
Disability certification in Nicaragua	**Population characteristics:** Population with disability. **WHODAS version used:** 36-item version. **Main findings:** Characterization and certification of disability using WHODAS 2.0. Identification of associated variables and verification of the usefulness of WHODAS 2.0 as an ICF-based tool in the local context (*48*).
Disability prevalence and characterization study in Panama	**Population characteristics:** National and subnational representative sample **WHODAS version used:** 36-item. **Main findings:** National and subnational disability prevalence were estimated. A questionnaire based on WHODAS was applied to the sample. A national atlas of disability was created with the results of this study (*49*).
Tsunami Recovery Impact Assessment and Monitoring System (TRIAMS)	**Population characteristics:** Household surveys in tsunami-affected areas of Indonesia (n = 10 859) and Thailand (n = 1190). **WHODAS 2.0 version used:** 12-item version. **Main findings:** Population in tsunami-affected areas showed worse level of functioning than general population norms. WHODAS 2.0 used as a health outcome indicator in tsunami-affected areas (*50*).

WHODAS 2.0 has proven useful in a wide range of clinical and service settings. Table 4.2 gives an overview of WHODAS 2.0 validation studies and different applications (e.g. measuring the functioning impact of different health conditions, identification of intervention needs and monitoring change over time).

Table 4.2 Clinical applications of WHODAS 2.0

Application name	Summary of application
Validation of WHODAS 2.0 in Italy	**Population characteristics:** People with and without disabilities. **WHODAS 2.0 version used:** 36-item version. **Main findings:** WHODAS 2.0 is a useful instrument for measuring disability and functioning. It has high reliability and a stable factor structure. Psychometric evaluation of a representative sample of Italian disabled people should be undertaken to reach standard scores for each macrocategory of disability (*51*).
Utility and feasibility of WHODAS 2.0 in mental and physical rehabilitation	**Population characteristics:** Patients with long-term physical and psychiatric illnesses in clinical rehabilitation. **WHODAS 2.0 version used:** 36-item version. **Main findings:** WHODAS 2.0 and WHO Quality of Life Brief Scale (WHOQOL-BREF) were found to be meaningful and feasible (*52*).
Validation of WHODAS 2.0 for patients with inflammatory arthritis	**Population characteristics:** Patients with early inflammatory arthritis. **WHODAS 2.0 version used:** 36-item version. **Main findings:** WHODAS 2.0 is a valid and reliable measure of health-related quality of life in cross-sectional studies. Research is still required to investigate potential item redundancy and determine its usefulness in longitudinal studies (*53*).
Validation of WHODAS 2.0 for patients with stroke	**Population characteristics:** Stroke patients and their closest others. **WHODAS 2.0 version used:** 36-item version. **Main findings:** WHODAS 2.0 is a reliable instrument for the assessment of stroke patients, both as a self-rating and an observer-rating questionnaire (*54*).
Validation of WHODAS 2.0 for patients with systemic sclerosis	**Population characteristics:** Patients with systemic sclerosis (SSc). **WHODAS 2.0 version used:** 36-item version. **Main findings:** WHODAS 2.0 had good psychometric properties in patients with SSc and should be considered a valid measure of health-related quality of life in SSc (*55*).
Disability levels of patients with depression before and after intervention	**Population characteristics:** Patients with depression. **WHODAS 2.0 version used:** 36-item version. **Main findings:** Levels of disability in patients with depression before and after receiving antidepressant treatment were identified (*52*).
Disability pattern in older community residents	**Population characteristics:** Older community residents in Nigeria. **WHODAS 2.0 version used:** 12-item version. **Main findings:** Patterns of disability and care were identified (*56*).
Validation of WHODAS 2.0 in Germany	**Population characteristics:** Patients with musculoskeletal diseases, internal diseases, stroke, breast cancer and depressive disorders. **WHODAS 2.0 version used:** 36-item version, in German. **Main findings:** Results support the usefulness, reliability, validity, dimensionality, and responsiveness of the instrument for measuring functioning and disability (*57*).
Health outcomes and return to work in patients with multiple injuries	**Population characteristics:** Prospective cohort study in patients with severe multiple injuries. **WHODAS 2.0 version used:** 36-item version. **Main findings:** WHODAS 2.0 disability scores in the studied population showed substantially worse functioning compared with general population data. Profession, injury severity, pain, and physical, cognitive and social functioning made independent contributions to WHODAS 2.0 two years after injury, and explained 69% of the variance of the model (*58*).
Validation of WHODAS 2.0 in Spain	**Population characteristics:** Different clinical populations. **WHODAS 2.0 version used:** 36-item, 12-item and 12+24-item version, in Spanish. **Main findings:** Description of the development of WHODAS 2.0 in Spain and other Spanish-speaking countries. Contains information and guidance on how to administer the different WHODAS 2.0 versions (in Spanish) (*59*).

Validation of WHODAS 2.0 for patients with anxiety disorders	**Population characteristics:** Outpatients with anxiety disorders. **WHODAS 2.0 version used:** 36-item version. **Main findings:** Compared with three other established generic effectiveness measures, WHODAS 2.0 was at least as sensitive as other generic effectiveness measures to changes in anxiety symptom, and was particularly sensitive to changes in social anxiety symptoms (*5*).
Validation of WHODAS 2.0 for patients with hearing loss	**Population characteristics:** Individuals with adult-onset hearing loss. **WHODAS 2.0 version used:** 36-item version. **Main findings:** WHODAS 2.0 communication, participation, and total scores can be used to examine the effects of adult-onset hearing loss on functional health status (*33*).
Disability levels and pattern in older Korean population	**Population characteristics:** Older Korean population. **WHODAS 2.0 version used:** 36-item version. **Main findings:** Level of disability, as measured by WHODAS 2.0, was principally associated with physical health, depression and cognitive function, rather than sociodemographic factors (*60*).
Utility and feasibility of WHODAS 2.0 in patients with long-term psychotic disorders	**Population characteristics:** Patients treated for long-term psychotic disorders. **WHODAS 2.0 version used:** 36-item version. **Main findings:** WHODAS 2.0 is a useful addition to clinician-rated measures for measuring the patient's own experience of disability (*61*).
Validation of WHODAS 2.0 for patients with schizophrenia in Turkey	**Population characteristics:** Patients with schizophrenia. **WHODAS 2.0 version used:** 36-item version. **Main findings:** Investigated the relation between symptoms and other patient characteristics and perceived stigmatization in patients with schizophrenia. Perceived stigmatization was measured by questions from WHODAS 2.0 (*62*).
Study of qualitative profiles of disability using WHODAS 2.0	**Population characteristics:** Clinical patients with spinal cord injury, Parkinson disease, stroke and depression. **WHODAS 2.0 version used:** 36-item version. **Main findings:** The identified profiles of functional disability are paralleled by increasing levels of disability (*63*).
Validation of WHODAS 2.0 for older patients with schizophrenia .	**Population characteristics:** Older patients with schizophrenia. **WHODAS 2.0 version used:** 36-item version. **Main findings:** Strong evidence for reliability and some evidence for validity of WHODAS 2.0 with these patients (*64*).
Disability assessment by general practitioners (GPs) in France	**Population characteristics:** Patients of five GPs in France. **WHODAS 2.0 version used:** 12-item version. **Main findings:** WHODAS 2.0 was found to be a useful instrument for depicting disability and service use in general practice (*65*).
Mental Health assessment by GPs in New Zealand	**Population characteristics:** Patients from a random sample of GPs in New Zealand. **WHODAS 2.0 version used:** 36-item version, self-administered. **Main findings:** GPs' assessment of the patients' psychological health corresponded with the patients' self-assessment of functioning (*66*).
Validation of HIV/AIDS specific measure	**Population characteristics:** HIV-infected patients. **WHODAS 2.0 version used:** 36-item version. **Main findings**: Convergent validity of the Multidimensional Quality of Life Questionnaire for HIV/AIDS (MQOL-HIV) with WHODAS 2.0 was satisfactory for most domains (*67*).
Validation of WHODAS 2.0 for patients with depression and low back pain	**Population characteristics:** Patients with depression and low back pain in primary care setting. **WHODAS 2.0 version used:** 36-item version. **Main findings:** WHODAS 2.0 had excellent internal validity and convergent validity in the primary care setting. The responsiveness to change of WHODAS 2.0 was comparable to that of SF-36 (*68–70*).

Utility and feasibility of WHODAS 2.0 in patients with ankylosing spondylitis (AS)	**Population characteristics:** Patients with AS. **WHODAS 2.0 version used:** 36-item version. **Main findings:** WHODAS 2.0 is a useful instrument for measuring disability in AS, because it accurately reflected disease-specific instruments and showed similar responsiveness scores. A short-term change on WHODAS 2.0 was found to be associated with a change in physical function (*71*).
WHODAS utilization in the National Rehabilitation Service (Argentina)	**Population characteristics:** 1100 patients with disability certified by the National Rehabilitation Service. **WHODAS version used:** 36-item and 12+24-item. **Main findings:** WHODAS 2.0 proved to be a useful instrument for measuring disability in the National Rehabilitation Service (*72*).

4.2 Further development of WHODAS 2.0

Impairment module

In selecting items for inclusion in WHODAS 2.0, impairment items were generally avoided, because they are largely disease specific. Nevertheless, some impairments are relatively common, and they require both assessment and special interventions. Many users have asked for the development of an additional module that covers impairments in body functions and structures.

A future WHODAS 2.0 impairment module could conceivably be derived from a selection of certain ICF impairment domains for use in general populations, as identified in Annex 9 of ICF (*2*). From this domain list, the impairment questions shown in Table 4.3 were developed and used in the MCSS and the World Health Surveys (*34,35*).

Table 4.3 Impairment questions used in the WHO Multi-Country Survey Study and the World Health Surveys

1	How much <u>bodily aches</u> or <u>pains</u> did you have?[a]
2	How much <u>bodily discomfort</u> did you have?
3	Have you had a problem with a <u>skin defect of face, body, arms or legs</u>?
4	Have you had a problem with your <u>appearance</u> due to <u>missing or deformed or paralyzed arms, legs, feet</u>?
5	How much difficulty did you have in <u>using your hands and fingers</u>, such as picking up small objects or opening or closing containers?
6	How much difficulty did you have in <u>seeing and recognizing a person you know across the road</u>? (Take into account eye glasses, if you wear them). *Read the text in brackets if you see respondent wearing glasses.*[b]
7	How much difficulty did you have in <u>seeing and recognizing an object at arm's length</u> or in reading? (Take into account eye glasses, if you wear them). *Read the text in brackets if you see respondent wearing glasses.*
8	How much difficulty did you have in <u>hearing someone talking on the other side of the room</u> in a normal voice? (Take into account hearing aids, if you use them). *Read the text in brackets if you see respondent using hearing aid.*
9	How much difficulty did you have in <u>hearing what is said in a conversation</u> with one other person in a quiet room? (Take into account hearing aids, if you use them). *Read the text in brackets if you see respondent using hearing aid.*
10	How much of a problem did you have <u>passing water</u> (urinating) or in controlling urine (incontinence)?
11	How much of a problem did you have with <u>defecating</u>, including constipation?
12	How much difficulty did you have with <u>shortness of breath at rest</u>?
13	How much difficulty did you have with <u>shortness of breath with mild exercise</u>, such as climbing uphill for 20 metres or stairs (such as 12 steps)?
14	How much difficulty did you have with <u>coughing or wheezing</u> for ten minutes or more at a time?
15	How much of the time did you have a problem with sleeping, such as: falling asleep, waking up frequently during the night or waking up too early in the morning?
16	How much of a problem did you have with <u>feeling sad, low or depressed</u>?
17	How much of a problem did you have with <u>worry or anxiety</u>?

[a] Underlining indicates emphasis.
[b] Italics indicates instructions for interviewer.

Environmental factors module

WHODAS 2.0 does not currently assess environmental factors. Assessment of a respondent's functioning includes enquiries about the current environment of the respondent, but coding is based on functioning and disability, not on the environment.

A module could be developed that would assess environmental factors and include enquiries into the impact of the environment on a person's functioning. This could be achieved, for example, by adding:

* additional probing questions to enquire about environmental factors where any difficulty is reported in the current WHODAS 2.0
* a new module on the environment as a whole, to assess the environment independently of WHODAS 2.0 domains.

Only the former approach was tried during the development field studies. It added to the complexity of the application and time of the interview, but some people found it useful. As a result, the WHO task force has decided to undertake it as a separate development project in a future version of WHODAS 2.0.

Clinician version

Clinicians do not generally like administering structured questionnaires, because the standardization requirements may alter the natural flow of a clinical encounter. The basic information can be captured in a more clinician-friendly assessment schedule that allows more flexibility but more in-depth enquiry options for clinicians. A good example of such an assessment style is the Schedules for Clinical Assessment in Neuropsychiatry (SCAN) (73). SCAN's basic feature is to define domains and items, while allowing the clinician to evaluate the presence and severity of those domains and items in the clinician's own style of interrogation.

Children and youth version

WHODAS 2.0 has basically been developed for adult populations. In field trials, it has been applied to young people aged over 12 years in some countries, but given the strict research criteria, at present, we cannot recommend its use in subjects below the age of 18 years.

In light of the growing importance of child and youth populations worldwide, and with the advent of the Children and Youth version of the ICF (ICF-CY), the need to assess functioning and disability in children and youth is becoming more prominent. WHO is therefore exploring the development of a children and youth version of WHODAS 2.0.

Linkage of WHODAS 2.0 to disability weights

Summary measures of population health combine data on disability with those on premature mortality to calculate the burden of disease for public health purposes. Given the importance of summary measures, one important application of WHODAS 2.0 has been to provide information on the extent of disability in different populations.

Epidemiological data on disability in populations with certain diseases are not available in certain parts of the world; therefore, producers of summary measures of population health have chosen to use other methods of estimation. The computation requires a value called "disability weight", also known as "preference" or "valuation" in econometrics. Different techniques are used to obtain estimates of this value from experts, people who have the disease or general populations.

WHODAS 2.0 is not a valuation instrument. The health state instruments can better be called "descriptors" of disability, whereas disability weight is a "valuation" of disability. These two constructs must be logically linked to arrive at better disability weights, instead of using complex estimation techniques. In this way, epidemiology of disability can empirically inform disability weights.

A WHO/NIH joint project included a supplement to explore this linkage (*74*). The research took place within the MCSS, in which WHODAS 2.0 was applied with other measures of valuation such as "visual analogue scale" and "time trade off" (*34*). The results show that, with proper regression techniques, WHODAS 2.0 could generate disability weights. Since valuation techniques require extensive interviews, this method is a good alternative to population surveys.

Part 2
Practical aspects of administering and scoring
WHODAS 2.0

5   Administering WHODAS 2.0

WHODAS 2.0 has been successfully administered in both population and clinical settings across a range of different cultures. This chapter presents generic information and instructions for the different modes of administering WHODAS 2.0, general guidelines for the application of the instrument and guidance on developing versions in different languages.

5.1   Access and conditions of use for WHODAS 2.0 and its translations

WHO is granting free access and use of WHODAS 2.0, and has therefore placed the instrument in the public domain. People wishing to use it can do so after completing an online registration form on the WHODAS 2.0 web site.[1] The information collected through the registration form is helping WHO to improve and share the knowledge base of WHODAS 2.0 applications and keep WHODAS 2.0 users up to date with the latest information and developments of the instrument.

Users of WHODAS 2.0 have no authority to make substantive changes to the assessment instrument unless given explicit permission to do so. Section 4.2 outlines the priority areas for future WHODAS 2.0 development. Users interested in contributing or supporting this work should contact WHO directly by e-mail.[2]

Currently, WHODAS 2.0 is available in the following languages: Albanian, Arabic, Bengali, Chinese (Mandarin), Croatian, Czech, Danish, Dutch, English, Finnish, French, German, Greek, Hindi, Italian, Japanese, Kannada, Korean, Norwegian, Portuguese, Romanian, Russian, Serbian, Slovenian, Spanish, Sinhala, Swedish, Tamil, Thai, Turkish and Yoruba.

WHO welcomes requests for translation of WHODAS 2.0 into other languages. Anyone interested in submitting such a request should do so by e-mail.[2]

5.2   Modes of administering WHODAS 2.0

There are three modes of administering WHODAS 2.0: self-administered, by interview and by proxy, each of which is discussed below.

5.2.1   Self-administration

A paper-and-pencil version of WHODAS 2.0 can be self-administered. All questions share similar stems, and the same timeframe and response scale. This gives the instrument a user-friendly, uncluttered and to-the-point style. Users are encouraged to photocopy the WHODAS 2.0 versions in Part 3 for research purposes.

5.2.2   Interview

WHODAS 2.0 can be administered in person or over the telephone. Again, the style is user friendly and avoids unnecessary repetitions. General interview techniques are sufficient to administer the interview in this mode. Chapter 7 contains question-by-question specifications that each interviewer must be trained in; training assistance is available through WHO. Chapter 10 contains a test that can be used to assess knowledge related to WHODAS 2.0.

5.2.3   Proxy

Sometimes it may be desirable to obtain a third-party view of functioning from someone other than the person being interviewed. For example, family members, caretakers or other observers may be asked to give their views on the domains of functioning formulated in WHODAS 2.0. Testing during field trials has shown that obtaining the views of a third party is useful.

---

[1]   http://www.who.int/whodas

[2]   Send e-mail to whodas@who.int

5.3   Training in the use of WHODAS 2.0

Standardization

WHODAS 2.0 interviews should be conducted in the same way with each participant. Such standardization helps to ensure that differences in participants' responses are not due to differences in the way the interview is conducted. For example, if an interviewer administers WHODAS 2.0 to certain participants in a group situation and to others alone, then differences in responses may be due solely to the different interview formats. The same principle holds for different interviewers. If one interviewer is friendly to participants and another is distant, then participants may give different types of responses. Clear training in standardized procedures helps to prevent these possibilities.

> This manual provides guidelines for standardized administration of WHODAS 2.0. Those administering the test should read the guidelines and follow them carefully. The key to success and the essence of standardization is to ensure that all versions of WHODAS 2.0 are administered in the same way each time they are used.

Privacy

Each participant must be given privacy. This ensures a high comfort level, which in turn gives the most accurate responses. For example, if WHODAS 2.0 is administered in a waiting room, there needs to be sufficient space between a participant and his or her neighbour to avoid the responses being seen by the neighbour. When WHODAS 2.0 is administered through an interview, this should be conducted in a closed room where responses cannot be overheard.

Frames of reference for answering questions

For all WHODAS 2.0 versions, respondents should answer questions with the following frames of reference in mind:

- frame 1 – degree of difficulty
- frame 2 – due to health conditions
- frame 3 – in the past 30 days
- frame 4 – averaging good and bad days
- frame 5 – as the respondent usually does the activity
- frame 6 – items not experienced in the past 30 days are not rated.

Interviewers should remind respondents about these frames of reference, as needed. The frames of reference are explained more fully below.

Frame of reference 1 – degree of difficulty

During the interview, respondents are asked questions about the degree of difficulty that they experience in doing different activities. For WHODAS 2.0, having difficulty with an activity means:

- increased effort
- discomfort or pain
- slowness
- changes in the way the person does the activity.

Frame of reference 2 – due to health conditions

Respondents are asked to answer about difficulties due to any health conditions, such as:

- diseases, illnesses or other health problems
- injuries
- mental or emotional problems
- problems with alcohol
- problems with drugs.

Interviewers should feel free to remind respondents to think about difficulty with activities due to health conditions, rather than to other causes. For example, item D3.1 of WHODAS 2.0 asks "How much difficulty did you have in washing your whole body?" The possible responses are as follows:

None	Mild	Moderate	Severe	Extreme or cannot do
1	2	3	4	5

If a respondent has difficulty with bathing simply because it is cold, the item would be rated "1" for none. However, if the respondent is unable to wash due to arthritis, the item would be rated "5" for extreme or cannot do.

Frame of reference 3 – in the past 30 days

Recall abilities are most accurate for the period of one month. The past 30 days was therefore selected as the timeframe for WHODAS 2.0.

Frame of reference 4 – averaging good and bad days

Some respondents will experience variability in the degree of difficulty that they experience over 30 days. In these cases, respondents should be asked to give a rating that averages good and bad days.

Frame of reference 5 – as the respondent usually does the activity

Respondents should rate the difficulty experienced by taking into consideration how they usually do the activity. If assistive devices or personal assistance are usually available, respondents should keep this in mind. For example, as mentioned above, item D3.1 asks "How much difficulty did you have in washing your whole body?", and possible responses again range from "None" to "Extreme or cannot do", or "Not applicable".

If a respondent with a spinal cord injury has a personal assistant who helps daily with bathing and therefore experiences no difficulty with washing his or her whole body because of the help available, the item would be rated "1" for "None". Interviewers who wish to evaluate the added value of personal or technical assistance are advised to ask the question twice (i.e. without and with personal or technical assistance). In the example of the respondent with a spinal cord injury, the item would be rated "1" (for "None") with help, but "5" (for "Extreme or cannot do") without help.

Frame of reference 6 – Items rated as not applicable

WHODAS 2.0 seeks to determine the amount of difficulty encountered in activities that a person actually does, as opposed to activities that the person would like to do or can do, but does not actually do. Interviewers should determine whether responses are applicable. For example, item D2.5 asks "How much difficulty did you have in walking a long distance, such as one kilometre?", and possible responses again range from "None" to "Extreme or cannot do", or "Not applicable".

If a respondent cannot walk one kilometre because he or she has a leg fracture, the item would be rated "5" for extreme or cannot do. However, if a respondent has not tried to walk one kilometre simply because he or she drives everywhere, then the item would be coded "N/A" for not applicable.

Another example is item D3.4, which asks "How much difficulty did you have in staying by yourself for a few days?", and possible responses again range from "None" to "Extreme or cannot do", or "Not applicable". If a respondent lives with her family and has not been alone for a few days in the past 30 days, the item would be coded "N/A" for "Not applicable".

6   Scoring of WHODAS 2.0

This chapter explains the scoring of WHODAS 2.0 short (12-item) and full (36-item) versions. The scoring of the full version of WHODAS 2.0 takes into account the paid-work status of the respondent, with 32 items being used if the respondent is not in gainful employment. The chapter also provides general population norms, to allow comparison of different individuals or groups against population standards derived from large international samples.

6.1   WHODAS 2.0 summary scores

There are two basic options for computing the summary scores for the WHODAS 2.0 short and full versions – simple and complex.

Simple scoring

In "simple scoring", the scores assigned to each of the items – "none" (1), "mild" (2) "moderate" (3), "severe" (4) and "extreme" (5) – are summed. This method is referred to as simple scoring because the scores from each of the items are simply added up without recoding or collapsing of response categories; thus, there is no weighting of individual items. This approach is practical to use as a hand-scoring approach, and may be the method of choice in busy clinical settings or in paper–pencil interview situations. Simple scoring of WHODAS is specific to the sample at hand and should not be assumed to be comparable across populations.

The psychometric properties of WHODAS 2.0 allow this additive calculation. In classical psychometric analysis (75), the WHODAS 2.0 structure has been shown to be unidimensional and to have high internal consistency (76). As a result, the simple sum of the scores of the items across all domains constitutes a statistic that is sufficient to describe the degree of functional limitations.

Complex scoring

The more complex method of scoring is called "item-response-theory" (IRT) based scoring; it takes into account multiple levels of difficulty for each WHODAS 2.0 item. This type of scoring for WHODAS 2.0 allows for more fine-grained analyses that make use of the full information of the response categories for comparative analysis across populations or subpopulations. It takes the coding for each item response as "none", "mild", "moderate", "severe" and "extreme" separately, and then uses a computer to determine the summary score by differentially weighting the items and the levels of severity. Basically, the scoring has three steps:

* *Step 1* – Summing of recoded item scores within each domain.
* *Step 2* – Summing of all six domain scores.
* *Step 3* – Converting the summary score into a metric ranging from 0 to 100 (where 0 = no disability; 100 = full disability).

The computer programme is available from the WHO web site;[1] it is also provided in Chapter 8 as SPSS syntax. This syntax can easily be transformed for other statistics packages. Any questions should be sent to WHO by e-mail.[2]

---

[1]   http://www.who.int/whodas
[2]   Send e-mail to whodas@who.int

6.2   WHODAS 2.0 domain scores

WHODAS 2.0 produces domain-specific scores for six different functioning domains –cognition, mobility, self-care, getting along, life activities (household and work) and participation. The items within these domains are presented in detail in Chapter 7. Users who would like to obtain WHODAS 2.0 domain scores need to use the full version (i.e. 36 items). The domain scores provide more detailed information than the summary score. They may be useful for comparing individuals or groups against one another or against population standards, and across time (e.g. before and after interventions or other comparisons).

All WHODAS 2.0 domain scores are calculated using either the simple or the IRT-based scoring method (*16*). However, in order to compare populations, the latter approach is more useful.

6.3   WHODAS 2.0 population norms

WHODAS 2.0 population norms were initially generated from two studies:

* A reliability and validity study (Wave 2, described in Section 2.3).
* The MCSS (*34*). This study was conducted in general population samples from 10 countries (China, Colombia, Egypt, Georgia, India, Indonesia, Mexico, Nigeria, Slovakia and Turkey). A subset of these data was used to derive the general population norms for WHODAS 2.0.

Together, these data sources yielded initial population norms for WHODAS 2.0. When new data are available, these norms will be updated periodically by WHO and published on the WHO web site.

Table 6.1 gives the population norms for IRT-based scoring of the WHODAS 2.0 full versions.

Figure 6.1 displays the similar information in graphic format. The figure shows that an individual with 22 positive item responses (x-axis: WHODAS 2.0 IRT based score) would correspond to the 80th percentile (y-axis: population percentile).

Table 6.1   **Population norms for <u>IRT-based scoring</u> of the WHODAS 2.0 <u>full version</u>**

Summary score	Population percentile
0	40.00
1	46.83
2	52.08
3	56.20
4	59.58
5	62.46
6	64.94
7	67.12
8	69.05
9	70.78
10	72.35
15	78.42
20	82.66
25	85.85
30	88.35
35	90.38
50	94.69
70	98.14
90	99.90
100	100.00

Figure 6.1   **Population distribution of <u>IRT-based</u> scores for WHODAS 2.0 – 36-item version**

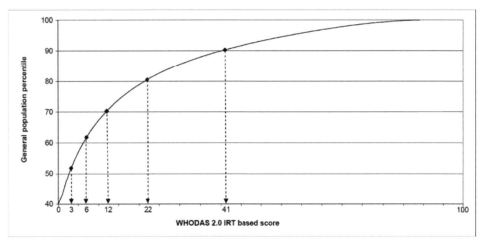

Source: *WHO Mutli-Country Survey Study on Health and Responsiveness 2000–2001(34)*

Table 6.2 shows the summary scores and population percentile for IRT-based scoring of the WHODAS 2.0 short version. Figure 6.2 summarizes the table graphically. The figure shows that an individual with a score of 17 (x-axis: WHODAS 2.0 IRT-based score) would correspond to the 90th percentile (y-axis: population percentile).

Table 6.2   **Population norms for <u>polytomous scoring</u> of the WHODAS 2.0 <u>short version</u>**

Summary score	Population percentile
0.0	50.0
2.8	63.2
5.6	73.3
8.3	78.1
11.1	82.0
13.9	86.5
16.7	89.6
19.4	92.4
22.2	93.0
25.0	93.8
27.8	94.7
30.6	94.9
41.7	97.2
58.3	99.7
100.0	100.0

Figure 6.2   **Population distribution of IRT-based score for WHODAS 2.0 – 12-item version**

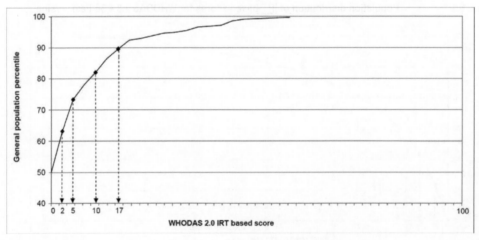

Source: *WHO Mutli-Country Survey Study on Health and Responsiveness 2000–2001(34)*

Population norms can be used in several ways. They provide values that can be used to compare different groups with each other, such as those with a diagnosis of physical problems to those with mental health problems. For example, to compare the degree of disability after a myocardial infarction with that due to severe depression, we recommend using the respective general population norms (i.e. percentiles) in the analysis.

6.4 WHODAS 2.0 item scores

In some instances, users may wish to compare items individually or by grouping some selected items of their choice. The WHODAS 2.0 raw item scores can be used as an ordinal scale that reflects the level of difficulty the respondent experiences in performing the particular function. The level of difficulty starts from "no difficulty" and increases in an ordered fashion to "mild", "moderate", "severe" or "extreme" difficulty. Each level indicates a higher degree of difficulty.

Like the overall summary score, the WHODAS 2.0 item scores could be used in two ways:

- *dichotomous (yes/no) scale* – indicating that the respondent has a difficulty in a particular domain of functioning, with the response scale for "mild", "moderate", "severe" and "extreme" all merged into a single positive coding; and

- *polytomous (multiple-level) scale* – which keeps the level of severity as it is; that is, as "mild", "moderate", "severe" or "extreme".

For item-level comparisons at individual level, the level of detail will require multiple level scoring. For larger groups, the dichotomous scoring may be used.

Item scores may be used in instances where frequencies of any difficulty for a given domain is to be reported.

6.5 Handling missing data within WHODAS 2.0

There are simple and complex ways of handling missing data in WHODAS 2.0; these are described below.

Simple approaches to missing data

We found that the following methods worked in experimental conditions, in large data sets, where it was possible to create artificial situations for missing data and recalculate the WHODAS 2.0 scales.

- For WHODAS 2.0 short version – The simplest approach, when only one item is missing a value, is to use the mean of the other items to assign a score to the missing item in the 12-item WHODAS 2.0. This method should not be used if more than one item is missing.

- For WHODAS 2.0 full version – The following approach is used where more than one item is missing:

    - If the respondent is not working and has given responses to the 32-item WHODAS 2.0, the score can be used as it is, and will be comparable to that of the full 36-item version.

    - In all other situations where one or two items are missing, the mean score across all items within the domain should be assigned to the missing items. This method should not be used if more than two items are missing. In addition, if domain-wise scores are being computed for domains, the two missing items should not come from the same domain.

Complex approaches to missing data

More complex approaches can be used by researchers working with large data sets where many other background variables are available. These methods need to be used also when either more than one or more than two items are missing in the 12-item and 36-item versions, respectively.

The first alternative is to use a "hot deck" imputation procedure. This procedure fills in missing item responses using observed values from similar (i.e. with common characteristics, such as age and sex) matched, randomly selected respondents with complete data from the same data set. The advantage of this procedure is that it preserves the distribution of the item values (77). Several alternative algorithms to implement this imputation procedure are available.

The second alternative is to use a multiple imputation procedure. Unlike "hot deck" imputation, which fills in a single value for each missing value, the multiple imputation procedure replaces each missing value with a set of plausible values that represent the uncertainty about the correct value to impute. These multiply imputed data sets – usually between 3 and 10 – are then analysed using standard procedures for complete data and the results combined from these analyses (78).

7 Question-by-question specifications

This chapter provides background information about what is intended by each question in WHODAS 2.0. Interviewers should use this information when respondents request clarification about specific questions and should **not offer their own interpretations.**

Each section from WHODAS 2.0 is listed alphabetically, based on the letter that precedes the question number. In this chapter, questions are shown in bold text, notes on what to record or why are given in plain text.

7.1 Questions A1–A5: Demographic and background information

This section should be completed with reference to the person completing the interview. A proxy should answer these questions with regard to the respondent.

A1	Record sex as observed
A2	How old are you now?
	Record age
A3	How many years in all did you spend <u>studying in school, college or university</u>?
	If the respondent dropped out of school or university, do not give credit for a partial year. If an individual has been in school both full- and part-time, note the number of years in full-time education. Count any repeated grades as two years.
A4	What is your <u>current marital status</u>?
	Allow the respondent to answer this question without reading the choices in advance. If the response does not correspond exactly with one of the provided responses, clarify by reading the choices that could correspond with the response.
	Select the option that best reflects current marital status. For example, if the respondent is currently married but was divorced in the past, score only currently married.
A5	Which describes your <u>main work status</u> best?
	Select the option that best reflects the respondent's current main work status. If doubtful about how to code a respondent (e.g. as homemaker or unemployed), rely on the respondent's judgement of their work status.
	There is no minimum number of hours per week that a respondent must work to qualify for the paid work category. Similarly, students need not be full time in order to be classed as such. In some versions, this item is used to determine whether respondents will be asked the series of work questions found in Domain 5. Therefore, if unsure about the response to this item, default to a category that will qualify the person to answer the questions about work in Domain 5.
	If the respondent reports being unemployed, ask: "is this for health reasons or for other reasons", and score accordingly.

7.2   Questions D1.1–D1.6: The six domains

Domain 1: Cognition

Domain 1 of WHODAS 2.0 asks questions about communication and thinking activities. Specific areas that are assessed include concentrating, remembering, problem solving, learning and communicating.

	In the past 30 days, how much difficulty did you have in:
D1.1	<u>Concentrating</u> on doing something for <u>ten minutes</u>?
	This question is intended to determine the respondent's rating of difficulty with concentration for a short period, defined here as 10 minutes. Generally, respondents understand this item. However, if clarification is requested, encourage the respondent to think about their concentration in usual circumstances, rather than when they are preoccupied by a problem or are in an unusually distracting environment. If necessary, prompt the respondent to think about their concentration while they were doing something such as work tasks, reading, writing, drawing, playing a musical instrument, assembling a piece of equipment, and so on.
D1.2	<u>Remembering</u> to do <u>important things</u>?
	This is a question about remembering matters of day-to-day importance. It does not refer to remembering irrelevant content or detailed information from the past. Ask respondents how well they remember to do things that are important to them or to their family. If a respondent normally uses some form of memory aid – for example, note-taking, electronic reminder systems or verbal cueing from personal assistants – then rate their performance with this aid taken into consideration.
D1.3	<u>Analysing and finding solutions to problems</u> in day-to-day life?
	This item refers to a complex activity involving many mental functions. If respondents are unsure of what the item means, ask them to think about a problem they encountered in the past 30 days. Once a problem is identified, respondents should be asked to consider how well they: • identified that a problem existed • broke it down into manageable parts • developed a list of possible solutions • determined the pros and cons of each solution • determined the best solution given all considerations • executed and evaluated the chosen solution • selected an alternate solution if the first choice was not successful.
D1.4	<u>Learning</u> a <u>new task</u>, for example, learning how to get to a new place?
	In this question, learning a new route is offered as an example. If respondents ask for clarification or appear to be thinking only about learning how to get to a new place, encourage them to think of other situations in the past month where learning something new was required, such as: • a task at work (e.g. a new procedure or assignment) • school (e.g. a new lesson) • home (e.g. learning a new home-repair task) • leisure (e.g. learning a new game or craft). Ask respondents, when rating themselves, to consider how easily they acquired new information, how much assistance or repetition they needed in order to learn and how well they retained what they learned.

D1.5	Generally understanding what people say?
	Ask respondents to consider their usual mode of communication (e.g. spoken language, sign language, use of an assistive device such as a hearing aid, etc.) and rate the overall degree of difficulty they have in understanding the messages of others. Respondents should consider all situations they have encountered in the past 30 days, such as: • when others spoke quickly • when there was background noise • when there were distractions. Difficulties due to different mother tongues should be excluded when rating this question.
D1.6	Starting and maintaining a conversation?
	Rate both starting and maintaining a conversation. If respondents state that they have more trouble starting than maintaining a conversation (or vice versa), ask them to average the amount of difficulty experienced with both activities to determine the final difficulty rating. Conversation includes use of whatever is the usual mode of communication (spoken, written, sign language, gestural). If respondents normally use assistive devices for communication, ensure that the difficulty rating provided takes into account conversation while using those devices. Ask respondents to consider any and all other factors related to a health condition and relevant to them in starting and maintaining a conversation. Examples might include hearing loss, language problems (e.g. as after a stroke), stuttering and anxiety.

Domain 2: Mobility

Activities discussed in Domain 2 of WHODAS 2.0 include standing, moving around inside the home, getting out of the home and walking a long distance.

	In the past 30 days, how much difficulty did you have in:
D2.1	Standing for long periods such as 30 minutes?
D2.2	Standing up from sitting down?
	This question refers to standing up from sitting in a chair, on a bench or a toilet. It does not refer to standing up from sitting on the floor.
D2.3	Moving around inside your home?
	This item refers to moving from room to room, and moving within rooms, using assistive devices or personal help that is usually in place. If a respondent lives in a house with multiple floors, this question also includes getting from one floor to another, as needed.
D2.4	Getting out of your home?
	This question seeks information about: • physical (mobility) aspects of getting out of the home • emotional or mental aspects of leaving the home (e.g. depression, anxiety, etc.) For this question, "home" means the respondent's current dwelling, which might be a house, apartment, or nursing home.
D2.5	Walking a long distance such as a kilometre [or equivalent]? [a]
	Convert distances into imperial measure where necessary (e.g. older people may be more familiar with miles than with kilometres).

[a] Square brackets [ ] contain instructions to translators

Domain 3: Self-care

Domain 3 asks about bathing, dressing, eating and staying alone.

		In the past 30 days, how much difficulty did you have in:
D3.1		Washing your whole body?
		This question refers to respondents washing their entire body in whatever manner is usual for their culture. If respondents report that they have not washed their bodies in the past 30 days, ask whether this is due to a health condition (as defined by WHODAS 2.0). If respondents report that it is due to a health condition, then code the item "5" for "Extreme or cannot do". If respondents report that the lack of washing is not due to a health condition, then code the item "N/A" for "Not applicable".
D3.2		Getting dressed?
		This question includes all aspects of dressing the upper and lower body. Ask respondents to consider activities such as gathering clothing from storage areas (i.e. closet, dressers) and securing buttons, tying knots, etc., when making the rating.
D3.3		Eating?
		This item refers to: • feeding oneself: that is, cutting food, and getting food or drink from a plate or glass to the mouth • swallowing both food and drink • mental or emotional factors that may contribute to difficulty in eating, such as anorexia, bulimia, or depression. This item does not refer to meal preparation. If a respondent uses non-oral feeding (e.g. tube feedings), this question refers to any difficulties experienced in self-administering the non-oral feeding; for example, setting up and cleaning a feeding pump.
D3.4		Staying by yourself for a few days?
		The intent of this question is to determine any difficulty respondents have in staying alone for an extended period and remaining safe. If respondents did not experience this situation in the past 30 days, "N/A" is the correct rating. If respondents give a rating of "None" for this question, probe the response to determine whether respondents stayed by themselves without difficulty (in which case "1" is correct) or whether they did not stay by themselves at all (in which case "N/A" is correct).

Domain 4: Getting along

Domain 4 assesses getting along with other people, and difficulties that might be encountered with this due to a health condition. In this context, "people" may be those with whom the respondent is intimate or knows well (e.g. spouse or partner, family members or close friends), or those whom the respondent does not know at all (e.g. strangers).

	In the past 30 days, how much difficulty did you have in:
D4.1	Dealing with people you do not know?
	This item refers to interactions with strangers in any situation, such as: • shop-keepers • service personnel • people from whom one is asking directions. When making the rating, ask respondents to consider both approaching such individuals, and interacting successfully with them to obtain a desired outcome.
D4.2	Maintaining a friendship?
	This item includes: • staying in touch • interacting with friends in customary ways • initiating activities with friends • participating in activities when invited. Respondents will sometimes report that they have not engaged in friendship-maintenance activities in the past 30 days. In this case, ask whether this situation is due to a health condition (as defined by WHODAS 2.0). If respondents report that it is due to a health condition, then code the item "5" for "Extreme or cannot do". If respondents report that it is not due to a health condition, then code the item "N/A".
D4.3	Getting along with people who are close to you?
	Ask respondents to consider any relationships that they define as close. These may be within or outside the family.
D4.4	Making new friends?
	This item includes: • seeking opportunities to meet new people • following up on invitations to get together • social and communication actions to make contact and to develop a friendship. On occasion, participants will report that they have not engaged in friendship-making activities in the past 30 days. In this case, interviewers should ask whether this is due to a health condition (as defined by the WHODAS 2.0). If respondents report that it is due to a health condition, then code the item "5" for "Extreme or cannot do". If respondents report that it is not due to a health condition, then code the item "N/A".
D4.5	Sexual activities?
	Ask respondents to think about what they consider to be sexual activities when answering this question. If asked for clarification, explain that this question refers to: • sexual intercourse • hugging • kissing • fondling • other intimate or sexual acts.

Domain 5: Life activities

This domain includes questions about difficulty in day-to-day activities. These activities are those that people do on most days; they include household, work and school activities. Ensure that flashcards #1 and #2 are visible.

Question-by-question specifications numbers in bold refer to the self-administered versions, and those in brackets refer to the interviewer-administered versions.

		Because of your health condition, in the past 30 days, how much difficulty did you have in:
D5.1		Taking care of your <u>household responsibilities</u>?
		This global question is intended to elicit respondents' appraisal of any difficulty they encounter in maintaining the household and in caring for family members or other people they are close to.
		Ask respondents to consider all types of household or family needs, including:
		• physical needs
		• emotional needs
		• financial needs
		• psychological needs.
		In some cultures, males may indicate that they do not have household responsibilities. In this situation, clarify that household responsibilities include:
		• managing finances
		• car and home repairs
		• caring for the outside area of the home
		• picking up children from school
		• helping with homework
		• disciplining children.
		Add any other examples that elucidate household responsibilities held by males in the culture, as necessary.
		Here, "household" is defined broadly. In the case of participants who do not have a stable dwelling place, there are still activities surrounding the upkeep and maintenance of their belongings. This question refers to those activities.
D5.2		Doing most important household tasks <u>well</u>?
D5.3		Getting all the household work <u>done</u> that you needed to do?
		Ask respondents to provide ratings based on their own appraisal of how well household tasks are completed and whether needed household work gets done. If necessary, remind respondents that they are to report only difficulties due to the health condition, not those that may be experienced for other reasons such as not having enough time (unless this reason is somehow linked to a health condition).
D5.4		Getting your household work done <u>as quickly</u> as needed?
		This question refers to the timely meeting of expectations and needs of those respondents whom one lives with (or is close to), in relation to household tasks and responsibilities.
D5.5		Your day-to-day <u>work/school</u>?
		This global question is intended to elicit respondents' appraisal of difficulties encountered in day-to-day work or school activities. This includes issues such as attending on time, responding to supervision, supervising others, planning and organizing, meeting expectations in the workplace and any other relevant activities.
D5.6		Doing your most important work/school tasks <u>well</u>?
		Doing work or school tasks "well" refers to completing them as expected by a supervisor or teacher, by respondents' own standards or as specified in the performance criteria for a job or school.

D5.7	Getting all the work <u>done</u> that you need to do?
D5.8	Getting your work done as <u>quickly</u> as needed?
	These questions refer to meeting work quantity expectations and time deadlines.

Domain 6: Participation

Domain 6 represents a shift from the line of questioning used in the first five domains. In this domain, respondents are asked to consider how other people and the world around them make it difficult for them to take part in society. Here, they are reporting not on their activity limitations but rather on the restrictions they experience from people, laws and other features of the world in which they find themselves. The underlined phrases in the introduction must be emphasized to help respondents shift their mindset and understand what is being asked. Respondents need to understand that the focus of these questions is on problems encountered because of the society in which they live rather than because of their own difficulties. This domain also includes questions about the impact of the health condition.

The introduction to this domain specifically reminds respondents that the focus of this interview is on the past 30 days. However, this particular domain does not readily lend itself to such a limited time frame; therefore, it is important to ask respondents to attempt to remain focused on the 30-day reference period.

	In the past 30 days:
D6.1	How much of a problem did you have <u>joining in community activities</u> (for example, festivities, religious or other activities) in the same way anyone else can?
	If necessary, clarify this question using other examples of community activities, such as attending town meetings, fairs, leisure or sporting activities in the town, neighbourhood or community. The relevant issue being asked in this question is whether respondents can participate in these activities or whether there are inhibitors to them doing so. If respondents appear confused by the phrase "in the same way anyone else can", ask them to use their judgement to: • assess the extent to which average people in their community can join community activities; and • consider their personal level of difficulty in joining community activities in relation to the assessment.
D6.2	How much of a problem did you have because of <u>barriers or hindrances</u> in the world around you?
	The intent of this question is to determine how much has stood in the way of respondents being able to realize aspirations and plans as other people can. The concept here is what respondents face in terms of external interference created by the world or other people. Barriers could be: • physical – for example, the lack of ramps to get into church; and • social – for example, laws that discriminate against people with disabilities and negative attitudes of other people that create barriers.
D6.3	How much of a problem did you have <u>living with dignity</u> because of the attitudes and actions of others?
	Ask respondents to consider problems they have had in living with dignity or pride in who they are, what they are doing and how they live their lives.

D6.4	How much <u>time</u> did <u>you</u> spend on your health condition, or its consequences?
	This question seeks to capture an overall rating or snapshot of the portion of the past 30 days spent by respondents in dealing with any aspect of their health condition. This may include time spent in activities such as:
	• visiting a treatment centre;
	• managing financial matters related to their health condition, such as payment of bills, reimbursement of insurance or benefits; and
	• obtaining information about the health condition or in educating others about it.
D6.5	How much have <u>you</u> been <u>emotionally affected</u> by your health condition?
	This question refers to the degree to which respondents have felt an emotional impact due to their health condition. Emotions may include anger, sorrow, regret, thankfulness, appreciation, or any other positive or negative emotions.
D6.6	How much has your health been a <u>drain on the financial resources</u> of you or your family?
	Family is broadly defined to include relatives; however, it also includes those to whom respondents are not related but consider to be like family, including those who may be sharing in the financial aspects of the health condition. The focus of this question is on the depletion of personal savings or current income to meet the needs created by a health condition. If respondents have experienced a significant financial drain but their family has not, or vice versa, they should respond to the question based on the drain experienced by either party.
D6.7	How much of a problem did your <u>family</u> have because of your health problems?
	The focus here is on problems created by the interaction of a respondent's health condition with the world in which the person lives. The question seeks information on problems that are borne by the family; these might include financial, emotional, physical problems, etc. The term "family" is defined above in D6.6.
D6.8	How much of a problem did you have in doing things <u>by yourself</u> for <u>relaxation or pleasure</u>?
	Ask respondents to consider leisure interests that they currently pursue and those they would like to pursue but cannot due to the health condition and restrictions imposed by society. Examples might include a respondent who:
	• would like to read novels but is restricted from doing so because the local library does not carry large-print books; and
	• enjoys watching movies but cannot do so because few are produced with subtitles for the deaf.
	Provide an overall rating of problems encountered.

7.3   Questions F1–F5: Face sheet

Questions F1–F7 are intended to gather demographic information about each respondent, and should be completed by the interviewer before the start of an interview.

F1	Record respondent or subject identification number.
F2	Record interviewer identification number.
F3	Record the assessment time point (time 1, time 2, etc.).
F4	Record the interview date in the format day/month/year, filling in blanks with zeros. For example, May 1st 2009 would be recorded as 01/05/09, not as 05/01/09.
F5	Indicate the respondent's living situation at the time of the interview. • 1 = Independent in community (i.e. living alone, with family, or friends in the community). • 2 = Assisted living (i.e. living in the community but receiving regular, professional assistance with at least some daily activities, such as shopping, bathing and meal preparation). • 3 = Hospitalized (i.e. residing in a 24-hour supervised setting such as a nursing home, hospital or rehabilitation facility).

7.4   Questions H1–H3: Effect of difficulties

Questions H1–H3 assess the extent to which the various difficulties respondents have encountered have affected their lives.

H1	Overall, in the past 30 days, how many days were these difficulties present?
	This is a global rating concerning all the difficulties assessed in the interview.
H2	In the past 30 days, for how many days were you totally unable to carry out your usual activities or work because of any health condition?
	Encourage respondents to use their own definitions of "totally unable" in answering this question.
H3	In the past 30 days, not counting the days that you were totally unable, for how many days did you cut back or reduce your usual activities or work because of any health condition?
	Ask respondents to consider any sort of reduction in usual activities, rather than counting only the days that they were totally unable to carry out activities.

7.5 Questions S1–S12: Short-form questions

Questions beginning with the letter "S" appear only in the 12-item and 12+24-item interviewer versions of WHODAS 2.0.

- In the 12-item version, all S items (S1–S12) are always asked.
- In the 12+24-item version, S1–S5 are always asked, but S6–S12 are asked only if the person has indicated some difficulty on the first five items.

	In the past 30 days, how much difficulty did you have in:
S1	Standing for long periods such as 30 minutes?
S2	Taking care of your household responsibilities?
	This global question is intended to elicit respondents' appraisal of any difficulty they encounter in maintaining the household and in caring for family members or other people they are close to. Ask respondents to consider all types of needs of the household or family, including needs that are: • physical • emotional • financial • psychological. In some cultures, males may indicate that they do not have household responsibilities. In this situation, clarify that household responsibilities include: • managing finances • car and home repairs • tending to the outside area of the home • picking up children from school • helping with homework • disciplining children. Add any other examples that elucidate household responsibilities held by males in the culture, as necessary. Here, "household" is defined broadly. In the case of participants who do not have a stable dwelling place, there are still activities surrounding the upkeep and maintenance of their belongings. This question refers to those activities.
S3	Learning a new task, for example, learning how to get to a new place?
	In this question, learning a new route is offered as an example. If respondents ask for clarification or appear to be thinking only about learning how to get to a new place, encourage them to think of other situations in the past month where learning something new was required, such as: • a task at work (e.g. a new procedure or assignment) • school (e.g. a new lesson) • home (e.g. learning a new home repair task) • leisure (e.g. learning a new game or craft). Ask respondents, when rating themselves, to consider how easily they acquired new information, how much assistance or repetition they needed in order to learn and how well they retained what they learned.

S4	<u>Joining in community activities</u> (for example, festivities, religious, or other activities) in the same way as anyone else can?
	If necessary, clarify this question using other examples of community activities, such as attending town meetings, fairs, leisure or sporting activities in the town, neighbourhood or community. The relevant issue being asked in this question is whether respondents can participate in these activities or whether their health condition inhibits them from doing so.
	If respondents appear confused by the phrase "in the same way as anyone else can", ask them to use their judgement to:
	• assess the extent to which average people in their community can join community activities; and
	• compare their degree of difficulty in joining community activities in relation to the assessment.
S5	How much have <u>you</u> been <u>emotionally affected</u> by your health problems?
	This question refers to the degree to which the respondent has felt an emotional impact due to the health condition. Emotions may include anger, sorrow, regret, thankfulness, appreciation, or any other positive or negative emotions.
S6	<u>Concentrating</u> on doing something for <u>ten minutes</u>?
	This question is intended to determine the respondent's rating of difficulty with concentration for a short period, defined as ten minutes. Generally, respondents have no problem understanding this item. However, if clarification is requested, encourage respondents to think about their concentration in usual circumstances, not when they are preoccupied by a problem situation or are in an unusually distracting environment. If necessary, prompt respondents to think about how difficult it was to concentrate while doing work tasks, reading, writing, drawing, playing a musical instrument, assembling a piece of equipment and so on.
S7	<u>Walking a long distance</u> such as a <u>kilometre</u> [or equivalent]?
	Convert distances into imperial measure where necessary.
	If respondents report that they have not walked this distance in the past 30 days, interviewers should ask whether this is due to a health condition (as defined by WHODAS 2.0). If respondents report that lack of walking is due to a health condition, then code the item "5" for "Extreme or cannot do". If respondents report that the lack of walking is not due to a health condition, then code the item "N/A" for "Not applicable".
S8	<u>Washing</u> your <u>whole body</u>?
	This question refers to respondents washing their entire body in whatever manner is usual for their culture.
	If respondents report that they have not washed their bodies in the past 30 days, ask whether this is due to a health condition (as defined by the WHODAS 2.0). If respondents report that it is due to a health condition, then code the item "5" for "Extreme or cannot do". If respondents report that the lack of washing is not due to a health condition, then code the item "N/A" for "Not applicable".
S9	Getting <u>dressed</u>?
	This question includes all aspects of dressing the upper and lower body. When making the rating, ask respondents to consider activities such as gathering clothing from storage areas (i.e. closet, dressers) and securing buttons, tying knots and so on.
S10	<u>Dealing</u> with people <u>you do not know</u>?
	This item refers to interactions with strangers in any situation, such as:
	• shop-keepers
	• service personnel
	• asking someone for directions.
	When making the rating, ask respondents to consider both approaching such individuals, and interacting successfully with them to obtain a desired outcome.

S11	Maintaining a friendship?
	This includes: • staying in touch • interacting with friends in customary ways • initiating activities with friends • participating in activities when invited. Respondents will sometimes report that they have not engaged in friendship-maintenance activities in the past 30 days. In this case, ask whether this situation is due to a health condition (as defined by the WHODAS 2.0). If respondents report that it is due to a health condition, then code the item "5" for "Extreme or cannot do". If respondents report that it is not due to a health condition, then code the item "N/A" for "Not applicable".
S12	Your day-to-day work/school?
	This global question is intended to elicit respondents' appraisal of difficulties encountered in day-to-day work or school activities. This includes issues such as attending on time, responding to supervision, supervising others, planning and organizing, meeting expectations in the workplace and any other relevant activities.

8 Syntax for automatic computation of overall score using SPSS

The scoring algorithm listed below is available for download in SPSS format from the WHODAS 2.0 section of the WHO web site.[1]

Recode of polytomous items:

```
RECODE
D1_1
(1=0) (2=1) (3=2) (4=3) (5=4) INTO D11.
RECODE
D1_2
(1=0) (2=1) (3=2) (4=3) (5=4) INTO D12.
RECODE
D1_3
(1=0) (2=1) (3=2) (4=3) (5=4) INTO D13.
RECODE
D1_4
(1=0) (2=1) (3=2) (4=3) (5=4) INTO D14.
RECODE
D1_5
(1=0) (2=1) (3=1) (4=2) (5=2) INTO D15.
RECODE
D1_6
(1=0) (2=1) (3=1) (4=2) (5=2) INTO D16.
RECODE
D2_1
(1=0) (2=1) (3=2) (4=3) (5=4) INTO D21.
RECODE
D2_2
(1=0) (2=1) (3=1) (4=2) (5=2) INTO D22.
RECODE
D2_3
(1=0) (2=1) (3=1) (4=2) (5=2) INTO D23.
RECODE
D2_4
(1=0) (2=1) (3=2) (4=3) (5=4) INTO D24.
RECODE
D2_5
(1=0) (2=1) (3=2) (4=3) (5=4) INTO D25.
RECODE
D3_1
(1=0) (2=1) (3=1) (4=2) (5=2) INTO D31.
RECODE
D3_2
(1=0) (2=1) (3=2) (4=3) (5=4) INTO D32.
RECODE
D3_3
(1=0) (2=1) (3=1) (4=2) (5=2) INTO D33.
```

[1] http://www.who.int/whodas

RECODE
D3_4
(1=0) (2=1) (3=1) (4=2) (5=2) INTO D34.
RECODE
D4_1
(1=0) (2=1) (3=1) (4=2) (5=2) INTO D41.
RECODE
D4_2
(1=0) (2=1) (3=1) (4=2) (5=2) INTO D42.
RECODE
D4_3
(1=0) (2=1) (3=1) (4=2) (5=2) INTO D43.
RECODE
D4_4
(1=0) (2=1) (3=2) (4=3) (5=4) INTO D44.
RECODE
D4_5
(1=0) (2=1) (3=1) (4=2) (5=2) INTO D45.
RECODE
D5_2
(1=0) (2=1) (3=1) (4=2) (5=2) INTO D52.
RECODE
D5_3
(1=0) (2=1) (3=1) (4=2) (5=2) INTO D53.
RECODE
D5_4
(1=0) (2=1) (3=2) (4=3) (5=4) INTO D54.
RECODE
D5_5
(1=0) (2=1) (3=1) (4=2) (5=2) INTO D55.
RECODE
D6_1
(1=0) (2=1) (3=1) (4=2) (5=2) INTO D61.
RECODE
D6_2
(1=0) (2=1) (3=2) (4=3) (5=4) INTO D62.
RECODE
D6_3
(1=0) (2=1) (3=1) (4=2) (5=2) INTO D63.
RECODE
D6_4
(1=0) (2=1) (3=2) (4=3) (5=4) INTO D64.
RECODE
D6_5
(1=0) (2=1) (3=2) (4=3) (5=4) INTO D65.
RECODE
D6_6
(1=0) (2=1) (3=1) (4=2) (5=2) INTO D66.
RECODE
D6_7
(1=0) (2=1) (3=2) (4=3) (5=4) INTO D67.

RECODE
D6_8
(1=0) (2=1) (3=1) (4=2) (5=2) INTO D68.
RECODE
D5_8
(1=0) (2=1) (3=1) (4=2) (5=2) INTO D58.
RECODE
D5_9
(1=0) (2=1) (3=2) (4=3) (5=4) INTO D59.
RECODE
D5_10
(1=0) (2=1) (3=2) (4=3) (5=4) INTO D510.
RECODE
D5_11
(1=0) (2=1) (3=2) (4=3) (5=4) INTO D511.

For summary scores of domains (do), where domain 1 is abbreviated as Do1, domain 2 as Do2, etc.

compute Do1 = (d11+d12+d13+d14+d15+d16)*100/20.
compute Do2 = (d21+d22+d23+d24+d25)*100/16.
compute Do3 = (d31+d32+d33+d34)*100/10.
compute Do4 = (d41+d42+d43+d44+d45)*100/12.
compute Do51 = (d52+d53+d54+d55)*100/10.
compute Do52 = (d58+d59+d510+d511)*100/14.
compute Do6 = (d61+d62+d63+d64+d65+d66+d67+D68)*100/24.

For summary score of WHODAS 2.0 without the remunerated work items:

compute
st_s32=(D11+D12+D13+D14+D15+D16+D21+D22+D23+D24+D25+D31+D32+D33+D34+D41
+D42+D43+
D44+D45+D52+D53+D54+D55+D61+D62+D63+D64+D65+D66+D67+D68)*100/92.

For summary score of WHODAS 2.0 with the remunerated work items:

compute
st_s36=(D11+D12+D13+D14+D15+D16+D21+D22+D23+D24+D25+D31+D32+D33+D34+D41
+D42+D43+D44+D45+D52+D53+D54+D55+D58+D59+D510+D511+D61+D62+
D63+D64+D65+D66+D67+D68)*100/106.

9   Guidelines and exercises for use of WHODAS 2.0

This chapter is intended for those administering WHODAS 2.0. Readers should first read Chapter 5 (Section 5.3), which explains the importance of both standardization and privacy in gathering data from questionnaires. Chapter 5 also provides background information on the frames of reference for answering questions.

Objectives

After reading the subsection on frame of reference for answering in Chapter 5 (Section 5.3), you will be able to:

- state the six points respondents should take into consideration while answering the WHODAS 2.0 questions; and
- distinguish between "Extreme or cannot do" and "Not applicable" answers.

9.1   Interviewer-administered version specifications

This section pertains only to the interviewer-administered versions, and contains information specific to these versions, including interviewer-administered proxy versions.

Objectives

After reading this section on general interviewing instructions, you will be able to:

- identify key features of good interviewing technique;
- list the key points to review during an interview introduction; and
- state two reasons for giving respondents feedback during the interview.

As you prepare to administer WHODAS 2.0, it is useful to review some general points about interviewing.

Keep the following points in mind:

- Be serious, pleasant, and self-confident; nervousness can make the respondent feel uneasy.
- Speak slowly and clearly to set the tone for the interview.
- Appear interested in the research.
- Be aware that different respondents require different amounts of information about the study, and adjust your introductions accordingly.

Some of these points are discussed below.

Make a good introduction

A good introduction to an interview is essential. It communicates the goals of the interview and sets the tone of the interaction. Be sure to make clear in your introduction:

- your name and professional affiliation;
- that you are a professional interviewer or clinician;
- that you represent a legitimate and reputable organization;
- that the questionnaire is for gathering information for important, worthwhile research;
- that the respondent's participation is vital to the success of the research; and
- that responses will be kept confidential to the extent provided for by law or by site-specific regulations.

Provide feedback as necessary

To give feedback, use neutral phrases in reaction to the respondent's behavior throughout the interview. Feedback is an effective tool for maintaining control over the interview. It can be used to:

- reinforce focused, attentive respondent behavior; and
- discourage digression, distraction and inappropriate enquiries.

When respondents have inappropriate enquiries (e.g. asking for advice, information or the interviewer's personal experiences), use one of these phrases:

- "In this interview, we are really interested in learning about your experiences."
- "When we finish, let's talk about that."
- "We will come to that later."

When respondents digress from the questions by giving lengthy responses or providing more information than is necessary, use one of these phrases:

- "I have many more questions to ask, so we should move on to those now."
- "If you would like to talk more about that we can do that at the end of the interview."

These two sentences are very effective when used together. Silence also can be an effective tool for discouraging inappropriate responses or conversation.

9.2   Typographical conventions

Objectives

After reading this section on typographical conventions, you will be able to:

- identify and properly use interviewer instructions located throughout WHODAS 2.0; and
- know the meaning of different typefaces (blue; bold and italics; underlined), parentheses (brackets) and square brackets.

The interviewer-administered versions use the typographical conventions listed below. Refer to WHODAS 2.0 as you read through this section, to ensure that you are familiar with these rules.

1   Interviewer instructions

Anything written in standard print in blue is meant to be read to the respondent. Anything written in bold and italics is an interviewer instruction and should not be read aloud.

Example:

B2 How do you rate your physical health in the past 30 days?

(Read response scale to respondent)

In this case, the interviewer would read aloud the response scale.

2 Skips within questions

"Skip instructions" are printed in bold and italics. Skips are automatically programmed into the computer version.

Example:

Before D5.7:

If box is checked, continue, otherwise, skip to Domain 6 on the next page.

3 Underlined type

Within questions, words in <u>underlined</u> typeface are key words or phrases that are to be emphasized when read to the respondent.

4 Verbatim entries

A blank line or blank computer field is provided when the interviewer is to record the respondent's answer.

Responses should be recorded exactly as stated.

This type of response is requested when further detail is needed:

Example:

A5 Which describes your main work status best?

(Select the single best option)

Choice 9 Other (specify) _____

5 Parentheses

Parentheses ( ) contain examples to illustrate a point.

All items in the parentheses are to be read to the respondent.

Example:

S4 How much of a problem did you have <u>joining in community activities</u> (for example, festivities, religious or other activities) in the same way as anyone else can?

In this case, the interviewer would read aloud the text in parentheses.

6 Square brackets

Square brackets [ ] contain instructions to translators. English-speaking interviewers may also follow these guidelines if needed to increase the clarity of the question or the applicability in the respondent's culture.

Example:

D2.5 Walking a long distance such as a kilometre [or equivalent]

9.3   Using flashcards

Objective

After reading this section on flashcards, you will be able to:

• identify and properly use the two WHODAS 2.0 flashcards.

Two flashcards are used in WHODAS 2.0 interviewer versions. The purpose of the flashcards is to provide a visual cue or reminder to the respondent about important pieces of information to remember while answering questions. Review the flashcards as you read through this section.

Flashcard #1 is the first card to be used in the interview. It provides information about how "health conditions" and "having difficulty" are defined, and reminds the respondent that the timeframe for evaluation is the past 30 days. The information on this card provides the respondent with useful reminders throughout the interview.

Flashcard #2 is the second card to be used in the interview. It provides the response scale to be used for most questions. When introducing this scale, you should read aloud the number and the corresponding word. Respondents may either point to their answer on the scale or provide responses verbally, although the latter is preferred.

• Ensure that flashcards #1 and #2 are visible to the respondent at all times during the interview.

• Follow the interviewer instructions provided throughout the instrument, which note when each flashcard should be pointed out to the respondent.

9.4   Asking the questions

Objective

After reading this section on how to ask WHODAS 2.0 questions, you will be able to:

• use the standardized method for asking questions of respondents.

Read the questions in their entirety and in the order they appear to ensure comparability across respondents. Even slight deviations from wording and the ordering of questions can affect responses.

1   Read questions as they are written

Read questions to the respondents exactly as they appear in the questionnaire. There are two exceptions to this rule in the administration of WHODAS 2.0 – grammatical changes and verifying responses – described below

Grammatical changes

If necessary, adjust the wording of a question to make it grammatically correct. This mainly occurs when only one difficulty is identified in a domain.

Example:

• In response to the question "How much did these difficulties <u>interfere</u> with your life?" if a respondent indicates only one difficulty in the domain, change the word "difficulties" to the singular "difficulty" and "these" to "this."

Verifying responses

If necessary, modify the form of the word used in the rating scale to make better sense.

Example:

- In response to the question "How much have you been emotionally affected by your health condition?" the answer "none" would be odd and grammatically incorrect. In this case, "none" can be changed to "not at all" to be grammatically correct. Many respondents make this shift automatically but the interviewer can provide guidance if necessary.

2   Read the entire question

Before accepting an answer, make sure that the respondent has heard the entire question, to ensure that the person is considering all concepts in the question. If the respondent interrupts before hearing the whole question, repeat the question, making sure that the respondent hears it through to the end. Do not assume that a premature response applies to the question as written.

3   Use lead-in phrases

The phrase "how much difficulty did you have in …" is used frequently throughout the interview. Repeat this phrase more or less frequently, as necessary, to help the respondent to complete the interview or to make the line of questioning flow more smoothly.

4   Use flashcards where instructed

Most questions use flashcards to remind the respondent of key information. The text *(point to flashcard #)* appears at each point where a flashcard is to be shown.

Do not make assumptions about the respondent's answers. Interviewers often develop a strong sense of the lifestyle or health condition of a respondent early in the interview and become convinced that answers to some questions will be negative. It is tempting to skip those questions or to introduce them with a phrase like "I know this probably doesn't apply to you, but …" Practices such as these make it impossible to get accurate information or to learn to what extent answers to earlier questions actually do predict answers to later ones. Avoid making assumptions and avoid the bias toward negative answers created by interjecting such comments.

9.5   Clarifying unclear responses

> **Objective**
>
> After reading this section on clarifying unclear responses, you will be able to:
>
> - use the standardized methods for clarifying and probing.

Clarification is required when a respondent is unable to answer a question because he or she does not understand all or some part of the question.

Probing is required when the respondent appears to understand the question and yet offers a response that does not meet the objective of the question. When this occurs, use non-directive probing or repeat the questions.

1   Rules for clarification and probing

(a) If you doubt that respondents heard the entire question, repeat it. For example, if respondents answer irrelevantly or do not appear to understand all aspects of the question, re-read either the whole question or the portion that was not understood.

(b) When respondents ask about a specific part of the question, repeat only that part.

(c) When asked to repeat one response option, repeat all response options, only omitting a response option if respondents have already clearly eliminated that option.

(d) Use only the question text or neutral probes to avoid introducing bias into the question.

(e) In repeating a question, it is sometimes helpful to use a neutral introduction to make a smoother transition; for example, preface the repeated question with:

- *Overall …*

- *Let me repeat the question …*

- *Well, in general …*

- *Generally speaking …*

(f) If respondents ask for clarification about what is being asked, first simply repeat the question. If respondents do not find this approach helpful, use the explanations as they are written in the question-by-question specifications given in Chapter 7; do **not** use any other definition of terms or explanations.

(g) If respondents request a definition for a term or an explanation that is not in the question-by-question objectives, instruct them to answer the question using their own definition or interpretation of the word, phrase or concept in question. To do this, use phrases such as:

- *Whatever ... means to you.*

- *Whatever you think of as ....*

2   Types of probes

Use neutral probes as necessary to help respondents provide descriptions when requested as part of the interview (i.e. *Please describe*) or to arrive at a single response. Questions that use the rating scale should have only one answer circled. Examples of suitable neutral probes include:

- *Can you tell me what you mean by that?*
- *Can you tell me more about that?*
- *What do you think?*
- *Which would be closer – slight or moderate?*
- *Can you think of any others?*
- *What is your best estimate?*
- *Can you be more specific?*
- *Can you give me your best guess?*
- *Can you provide one overall rating?*

3   Common probing situations

The following are common situations that require probing in WHODAS 2.0.

Don't know

The general rule when respondents give a response of "I don't know" is to repeat the question. If this is unsuccessful, probe respondents once before accepting the "don't know" (DK). An effort at recall should be encouraged with a probe such as "Could you give me your best estimate?" If respondents still cannot respond, "DK" is recorded in the left margin. The computerized version of the instrument provides a DK response category.

Not applicable

Respondents may sometimes feel that a question does not apply to their situation; for example, where they did not encounter the situation being queried (e.g. for question D4.5, regarding sexual activities). In this case, record the item with N/A in the left margin or with the N/A response choice in the computer version.

Probe all responses of "not applicable". If, in the process of probing, it appears that respondents feel a question is not applicable because they cannot do the activity, score the item as a "5" on the scale "cannot do." An appropriate probe in this situation would be:

*   *Can you tell me why this question does not apply to you?*

Reasons given by respondents may include issues such as the activity not being expected of them in their culture, or the activity not having been experienced in the past 30 days.

Discrepancies

Look out for discrepant responses. Refer respondents back to information on the flashcards as often as necessary if it seems that such information is being forgotten. For example, where respondents are clearly answering questions, but are indicating difficulties for reasons other than the health condition. It can be helpful to use the information on the flashcards as a reminder, but avoid engaging in confrontation or open ended probing to resolve perceived discrepancies.

9.6   Recording data

> **Objective**
>
> After reading this section on recording data, you will be able to:
>
> *   properly complete WHODAS 2.0 interview forms.

Do not use red ink or a red pencil when recording data. Print answers to all open-ended responses clearly using block letters.

Closed questions

Write or type all answers in the spaces provided.

Circling answer

Most questions require that an answer be circled. Make sure that the circle encloses only one number, because the computer will allow only one response selection.

Interviewer corrections

If an incorrect answer is circled because respondents change their mind or you make a mistake, put a slash (/) through the incorrect answer and circle the correct answer or write it in above. Answers can easily be corrected in the computer version of the instrument.

Fill-in codes

Some answers require entry of a number; in this case "right-justify" the answers.

Example:

A3 How many years in all did you spend studying in school, college or university?

The response "Nine years" would be written as "09 years".

Margin notes

Qualified responses to closed questions

A qualified response is one in which respondents give a codable response, but temper their answer with conditional descriptions such as "if," "except" or "but". Code such answers, and record the qualifications in the left margin of the form, because such comments may provide information that is important to the researchers.

Continue to follow the skipping pattern as indicated for the coded response. Sometimes, respondents will simply explain their responses rather than qualify them. Explanations are often signaled by words such as "because," "when," or sometimes by the use of a synonym for the response. Do not record such respondent comments in the margins.

Uncertainty about respondent's answer

If uncertain about a respondent's answer, repeat the question and record the answer exactly (i.e. when in doubt, do not paraphrase a response). If clear about a response but unsure about how to code it, record enough information in the left margin to allow the principal investigator or study coordinator to make a decision. Also use a question mark (?) in the left margin to indicate the uncertainty to the principal investigator or study coordinator.

Missing data

Missed questions

If a question is accidentally missed during the interview, enter "MISSED" in the left margin of the form. This indicates to the editor that the question was not asked.

If a missed question is noticed during an interview, go back and ask the question, making a note in the margin that the question was asked out of sequence.

If a missed question is only discovered after the interview, decide whether to recontact the respondent or accept the missing data. The computer-administered version will not allow the interview to progress if a question is not answered.

Refusal to answer

Always record refusals to answer questions, by writing "REFUSED (RF)" in the left margin or in the blanks provided for recording the response. When using the computerized version of the instrument, score refused questions as "don't know." If there is a refusal to respond to an open-ended question when using the computerized version, type "respondent refused" in the field provided for the answer.

Skipped questions

Questions skipped due to the skip rules should be left blank. Skips built into the computer version will automatically bypass questions.

Post-interview editing

When conducting an interview, there may be times when it is necessary to compromise data recording to maintain the flow of the interaction. To ensure that all data are recorded in a way that is meaningful, clear and readable to the researchers, edit the recorded data as necessary after the interview, as described below.

- Shortly after finishing each interview – and before starting the next – thoroughly check that all questions were completely and legibly answered. Where possible, do this while the respondent is present so that the person can help in correcting any omissions, if necessary.

- During post-editing, enter "MISSED" in the left margin next to any question that was unintentionally skipped during the interview.

- Turn completed interviews in to the study supervisor promptly, no less than once a week, so that any errors in administration can be noted and procedures corrected before further interviews are conducted.

9.7   Problems and solutions

A list of common problems found in administering WHODAS 2.0 and the solutions to these problems is given below.

Problem
I am having difficulty knowing when to code "not applicable" and when to code "cannot do."

Solution

WHODAS 2.0 seeks to determine the amount of difficulty encountered in activities that respondents actually do as opposed to activities they would like to do or those they can do, but don't.

If a respondent is prevented from doing an activity due to a health condition, rate the item as "5" for "Extreme or cannot do".

If a respondent has not experienced an activity in the past 30 days, but this is not due to a health condition, code the item as "N/A" for "Not applicable".

Problem
The respondent gives an answer that does not correspond with my (or others) understanding of the respondent's current functioning.

Solution

WHODAS 2.0 measures responses from the perspective of the respondent or – in the case of proxy versions – from a proxy respondent referring to the primary respondent's functioning. Although an interviewer might not always agree with the respondent's answer, the answer given must be the one recorded. This may be frustrating, but researchers must follow this standard to provide consistency in administration of the instrument.

Problem
The respondent does not give a clearly codable answer.

Solution

If the respondent does not give clear answers, probe the respondent for further clarification.

Problem
The respondent becomes annoyed by repetitious questions.

Solution

Some of the WHODAS 2.0 questions sound similar. In some cases, the respondent may become annoyed and assume that the interviewer was not listening to a previous response. In this situation, the interviewer has two options:

- **Ask the question with a preface** – that is, read the question with a preface that acknowledges previous responses; for example

  - "You told me before that...., but I still need to ask you this question as it is written."

- **Confirm the response** – that is, reword the question in a way that confirms the information that the respondent already gave; for example

  - "You told me before that....Is that correct?"

10 Test yourself

This chapter allows readers to complete a final review of the material covered in this training manual. Complete the questions, and turn to page 78 of this manual to check your answers. Next to each answer in parentheses is the section that provides the information from which the answer is derived. If you answer a question incorrectly, return to the section indicated and re-read that portion of the training manual. The more thoroughly you know the material contained within the training manual, the easier it will be to implement WHODAS 2.0.

10.1 Questions

1. A respondent has not walked one kilometre in the past 30 days due to a leg fracture, this item would be coded as:

    ❑ a. "Extreme or cannot do"

    ❑ b. "Not applicable"

2. A respondent has a spinal cord injury, and is unable to wash her body on her own. However, she usually has the help of a personal assistant, and has no difficulty washing her body with this assistance. The difficulty of this activity would be coded as:

    ❑ a. "Extreme or cannot do"

    ❑ b. "None"

3. In interviewer-administered versions of the WHODAS 2.0, anything written in standard print is meant to be read to the respondent.

    ❑ a. True

    ❑ b. False

4. The interviewer must read aloud each example contained in parentheses to illustrate the point.

    ❑ a. True

    ❑ b. False

5. A respondent can either point to his answer on a flashcard, or may provide responses verbally.

    ❑ a. True

    ❑ b. False

6. If a respondent interrupts the interviewer before hearing the whole question, the interviewer must repeat the question from the beginning.

    ❑ a. True

    ❑ b. False

7. If a respondent asks about a specific part of a question, the entire question should be repeated.

    ❑ a. True

    ❑ b. False

8. If a respondent gives a response of "I don't know", and a probing question does not elicit another response, the interviewer should then record the original answer.

    ❑ a. True

    ❑ b. False

9. Interviewers can use open-ended probing to resolve perceived discrepancies in a respondent's answers.

    ❑ a. True

    ❑ b. False

10. If a respondent gives an answer that does not correspond with the interviewer's understanding of the respondent's current functioning, the answer recorded should be:

    ❑ a. The respondent's version

    ❑ b. The interviewer's version

11. If a person is unable to report on his own difficulties, a proxy report can be used. In this case, the proxy should complete the:

    ❑ a. Self-report version, answering how they perceive the primary respondent would respond

    ❑ b. Proxy version, providing his or her own perceptions

12. In WHODAS 2.0, "health conditions" include physical and mental illnesses, as well as alcohol and drug problems.

    ❑ a. True

    ❑ b. False

13. Standardization means that you administer the interview using the same procedures every time.

    ❑ a. True

    ❑ b. False

14. In WHODAS 2.0, health conditions include physical and mental illnesses, injuries, but not alcohol or drug problems.

    ❑ a. True

    ❑ b. False

15. Respondents should answer questions taking into account the degree of difficulty they experience _____ the use of assistive devices or personal assistants.

   ❑ a. with

   ❑ b. without

16. Respondents should answer questions taking into account the worst day(s) they have experienced in the past 30 days.

   ❑ a. True

   ❑ b. False

17. A respondent answers that she has not attempted to learn new tasks in the past 30 days. Upon probing by the interviewer, she clarifies that this is not due to a health condition. This response should be rated:

   ❑ a. Not applicable

   ❑ b. Extreme or cannot do

18. The date is to be written in the European format of day/month/year.

   ❑ a. True

   ❑ b. False

19. When making your introduction, be sure to state (check two):

   ❑ a. The purpose of the evaluation

   ❑ b. That information will be kept confidential

   ❑ c. The similar types of problems you have experienced in your own life

20. As a general rule, it is a good idea to speak more rapidly than usual so you can finish the interview as quickly as possible.

   ❑ a. True

   ❑ b. False

21. When respondents provide more information than seems necessary:

   ❑ a. Make a careful note of the comments in the margin

   ❑ b. Tell the participant that you have many more questions to ask

22. In WHODAS 2.0, anything written in standard print is meant to be read to the respondent.

   ❑ a. True

   ❑ b. False

23. Text written in parentheses should be read only if respondents request clarification.

  ❏ a. True

  ❏ b. False

24. Text underlined should be emphasized to respondents.

  ❏ a. True

  ❏ b. False

25. It is important to introduce both flashcards at the beginning of the interview.

  ❏ a. True

  ❏ b. False

26. Once the flashcards are introduced, they should remain visible to the respondent throughout the interview.

  ❏ a. True

  ❏ b. False

27. In general, questions should be read to respondents exactly as they appear in the questionnaire.

  ❏ a. True

  ❏ b. False

28. If a respondent answers before you have read the entire question, you should:

  ❏ a. Accept the answer

  ❏ b. Read the remainder of the question

  ❏ c. Re-read the entire question

29. You should use the lead-in phrase "how much difficulty did you have in …"

  ❏ a. Before every question linked to this phrase

  ❏ b. More or less frequently to make the line of questioning flow smoothly

30. Probing is used when the respondent appears to understand the question, but does not provide a response that meets the objective of the question.

  ❏ a. True

  ❏ b. False

31. The interviewer must repeat all response options, even if the respondent asks the interviewer to just repeat one response option.

    ❑ a. True

    ❑ b. False

32. Neutral probes should be used rather than repeating the question text.

    ❑ a. True

    ❑ b. False

33. Interviewers can use the following to record data (check all that apply):

    ❑ a. Blue pen or pencil

    ❑ b. Red pen or pencil

    ❑ c. Black pen

    ❑ d. Green pen

    ❑ e. Pencil

34. When filling in blanks, answers should be "left-justified".

    ❑ a. True

    ❑ b. False

35. When a respondent clarifies a response with "because" or "when", the interviewer must record these answers in the margin.

    ❑ a. True

    ❑ b. False

36. As soon as an interviewer realizes that a question has been skipped, the interviewer must ask the missed question, and make a note in the margin stating that the question was asked out of sequence.

    ❑ a. True

    ❑ b False

10.2 Test yourself: Answers

1.a (Chapter 5 Section 5.3: Training in the use of WHODAS 2.0)	19.a, b (Chapter 9, Section 9.1: Interviewer-administered version specifications)
2. b (Chapter 5 Section 5.3: Training in the use of WHODAS 2.0)	20. b (Chapter 9, Section 9.1: Interviewer-administered version specifications)
3.a (Chapter 9, Section 9.2: Typographical conventions)	21.b (Chapter 9, Section 9.1: Interviewer-administered version specifications)
4.a (Chapter 9, Section 9.2: Typographical conventions)	22.a (Chapter 9, Section 9.2: Typographical conventions)
5.a (Chapter 9, Section 9.3: Using flashcards)	23.b (Chapter 9, Section 9.2: Typographical conventions)
6.a (Chapter 9, Section 9.5: Clarifying unclear responses)	24.b (Chapter 9, Section 9.2: Typographical conventions)
7.b (Chapter 9, Section 9.5: Clarifying unclear responses)	25.b (Chapter 9, Section 9.3: Using flashcards)
8.a (Chapter 9, Section 9.5: Clarifying unclear responses)	26.a (Chapter 9, Section 9.3: Using flashcards)
9.b (Chapter 9, Section 9.5: Clarifying unclear responses)	27.a (Chapter 9: Section 9.4: Asking the questions)
10.a (Chapter 9, Section 9.5: Clarifying unclear responses)	28.c (Chapter 9: Section 9.4: Asking the questions)
11.b (Chapter 5, Section 5.2: Modes of administrating WHODAS 2.0)	29.b (Chapter 9: Section 9.4: Asking the questions)
12.a (Chapter 5, Section 5.3: Training in the use of WHODAS 2.0)	30.a (Chapter 9, Section 9.5: Clarifying unclear responses)
13.a (Chapter 5, Section 5.3: Training in the use of WHODAS 2.0)	31.a (Chapter 9, Section 9.5: Clarifying unclear responses)
14.b (Chapter 5, Section 5.3: Training in the use of WHODAS 2.0)	32.b (Chapter 9, Section 9.5: Clarifying unclear responses)
15.a (Chapter 5, Section 5.3: Training in the use of WHODAS 2.0)	33.a,c,d,e (Chapter 9, Section 9.6: Recording data)
16.b (Chapter 5, Section 5.3: Training in the use of WHODAS 2.0)	34.b (Chapter 9, Section 9.6: Recording data)
17.a (Chapter 9, Section 9.7: Problems and solutions)	35.b (Chapter 9, Section 9.6: Recording data)
18.a (Chapter 7, Section 7.3: Questions F1–F7: Face sheet	36.a (Chapter 9, Section 9.6: Recording data)

Glossary

Activity

In the International Classification of Functioning, Disability and Health (ICF), the term "activity" is used in the broadest sense to capture the execution of a task or action by an individual at any level of complexity. It represents the individual's own perspective of their functioning. Activities include simple or basic physical functions of the person as a whole (e.g. grasping or moving a leg), basic and complex mental functions (e.g. learning and applying knowledge), and collections of physical and mental activities at various levels of complexity (e.g. driving a car, interacting with people). Other examples of activities include taking care of oneself and household work activities.

Activity limitations

Difficulties an individual may have in executing activities. An activity limitation encompasses all of the ways in which the execution of the activity may be affected; for example, doing the activity with pain or discomfort; too slowly or quickly, or not at the right time and place; awkwardly or otherwise not in the manner expected. Activity limitation may range from a slight to severe deviation (in terms of quality or quantity) in doing the activity, in a manner or to the extent that is expected of people without the health condition.

Assistive devices

All equipment or devices used by an individual to help with completion of an activity because of a health condition. Devices may be expensive (e.g. computers to aid communication) or simple (e.g. long-handled sponges for bathing).

Barriers or hindrances

External factors in a person's environment that, through their absence or presence, limit functioning and create disability. Includes aspects such as an inaccessible physical environment; lack of relevant assistive technology; negative attitudes of people towards disability; and services, systems and policies that are lacking or that hinder the involvement of all people with a health condition in any area of life.

Contextual factors

The complete background to a person's life and living, including external environmental factors and internal personal factors.

Difficulty

Experiencing discomfort, pain or slowness; needing to use increased effort; or having to make changes in the way an activity is done.

Disability

An umbrella term for impairments, activity limitations and participation restrictions. Denotes the negative aspects of the interaction between an individual (with a health condition) and that individual's environmental and personal context.

Environmental factors

Contextual factors that include the background of a person's life and living, composed of components of the natural environment (weather or terrain); the human-made environment (tools, furnishing, the built environment); social attitudes, customs, rules, practices and institutions, and other individuals.

Facilitators

Factors in a person's environment that, through their absence or presence, improve functioning and reduce disability. Includes aspects such as an accessible physical environment; availability of relevant assistive technology; positive attitudes of people towards disability; and services, systems and policies that aim to increase the involvement of all people with a health condition in all areas of life. Absence of a factor can also be facilitating (e.g. the absence of stigma or negative attitudes). Facilitators can prevent an impairment or activity limitation from becoming a participation restriction, since the actual performance of an action is improved, despite the person's problem with capacity.

Functioning

An umbrella term for body functions, body structures, activities and participation. Denotes the positive aspects of the interaction between an individual (with a health condition) and that individual's environmental and personal context.

Household activities

Activities involved with the physical, emotional, financial and psychological needs of the household or family. Includes tasks traditionally performed by men, such as managing finances, car and home repairs; caring for the outside area of the home; picking up children from school; helping with homework; and disciplining children.

Health condition

A disease that is short or long lasting; an injury (e.g. sustained in an accident); mental or emotional problems, which may range from stress due to day-to-day problems of living to more serious forms of mental illness; or problems with alcohol or drugs.

Impairment

Loss or abnormality in body structure or physiological function (including mental functions). "Abnormality" here strictly refers to a significant variation from established statistical norms (i.e. as a deviation from a population mean within measured standard norms) and should be used only in this sense. Examples of impairments include loss of an arm or leg or loss of vision. In the case of an injury to the spine, an impairment would be the resulting paralysis.

Participation

A person's involvement in a life situation. Represents the societal perspective of functioning.

Participation restrictions

Problems an individual may experience in involvement in life situations. Determined by comparing an individual's participation to that which is expected of an individual without disability in that culture or society.

Personal assistance

Any assistance from a person used to aid in the execution of an activity. May be paid or unpaid and may be completed by a family member or hired help. Personal assistance can take the form of actual physical help, or may involve verbal reminders, cues, prompts, presence, supervision or psychological help.

Personal factors

Contextual factors that include the background of a person's life and living, composed of features that are not part of a health condition or disability. Includes age, race, gender, educational background, experiences, personality and character style, aptitudes, other health conditions, fitness lifestyle, habits, upbringing, coping styles, social background, profession, and past and current experience.

Sexual activity

As assessed by WHODAS 2.0, sexual activity includes hugging, kissing, fondling, other intimate or sexual acts, and sexual intercourse.

References

1.   World Health Organization. *World health report 2000*. Geneva, WHO, 2000.

2.   World Health Organization. *International classification of functioning, disability and health (ICF)*. Geneva, World Health Organization, 2001.

3.   Üstün TB et al. *Disability and culture: universalism and diversity*. Seattle, Hogrefe & Huber Publishers, 2001.

4.   Üstün TB et al. World Health Organization Disability Assessment Schedule II (WHO DAS II): development, psychometric testing and applications. *Bulletin of the World Health Organization*, 2010, In press.

5.   Perini S, Slade T, Andrews G. Generic effectiveness measures: sensitivity to symptom change in anxiety disorders. *Journal of Affective Disorders*, 2006, 90(2–3):123–130.

6.   Harwood R et al. Measuring handicap: the London handicap scale, a new outcome measure for chronic disease. *Quality and Safety in Health Care*, 1994, 3(1):11–16.

7.   Ware J, Sherbourne C. The MOS 36-item short-form health survey (SF-36). I. Conceptual framework and item selection. *Medical Care*, 1992, 30(6):473–483.

8.   Ware J et al. *SF-36 health survey - manual and interpretation guide*. Boston, Massachusetts, Nimrod Press, 1993.

9.   Hays R, Prince-Embury S, Chen H. *RAND-36 health status inventory: manual*. San Antonio, McHorney, 1998.

10.   Jenkinson C, Fitzpatrick R, Argyle M. The Nottingham Health Profile: an analysis of its sensitivity in differentiating illness groups. *Social Science & Medicine*, 1988, 27(12):1411–1414.

11.   Hunt S et al. The Nottingham Health Profile: subjective health status and medical consultations. *Social Science & Medicine*, 1981, 15(3):221–229.

12.   Granger C et al. Performance profiles of the functional independence measure. *American Journal of Physical Medicine and Rehabilitation*, 1993, 72:84–89.

13.   Hobart J, Thompson A. The five item Barthel index. *Journal of Neurology, Neurosurgery & Psychiatry*, 2001, 71(2):225–230.

14.   Mahoney F, Barthel D. Functional evaluation: the Barthel index. *Maryland State Medical Journal*, 1965, 14:56–61.

15.   Kostanjsek N et al. Reliability of the World Health Organization disability assessment schedule - WHODAS II: subgroup analyses *(submitted for publication)*.

16.   Frick et al. Psychometric properties of the World Health Organization disability assessment schedule. *(WHO DAS II) (submitted for publication)*.

17.   Jablensky A et al. Schizophrenia: manifestations, incidence and course in different cultures. A World Health Organization ten-country study. *Psychological Medicine Monograph Supplement*, 1992, (20):1–97.

18.   Jablensky A, Schwarz R, Tomov T. WHO collaborative study on impairments and disabilities associated with schizophrenic disorders. A preliminary communication: objectives and methods. *Acta Psychiatrica Scandinavica*, 1980, 62(S285):152–163.

19.   Leff J et al. The international pilot study of schizophrenia: five-year follow-up findings. *Psychological Medicine,* 1992, 22(1):131–145.

20.   World Health Organization. *WHO psychiatric disability assessment schedule.* Geneva, WHO, 1988.

21.   Wiersma D, De Jong A, Ormel J. The Groningen Social Disabilities Schedule: development, relationship with ICIDH, and psychometric properties. *International Journal of Rehabilitation Research,* 1988, 11(3):213–224.

22.   Wiersma D et al. *GSDS-II - The Groningen Social Disabilities Schedule, second version.* Groningen, University of Groningen, Department of Social Psychiatry, 1990.

23.   Sartorius N, Üstün TB. The World Health Organization Quality of Life Assessment (WHOQOL): position paper from the World Health Organization. *Social Science & Medicine,* 1995, 41(10):1403–1409.

24.   Ziebland S, Fitzpatrick R, Jenkinson C. Tacit models of disability underlying health status instruments. *Social Science & Medicine,* 1993, 37(1):69–75.

25.   Andrews G, Peters L, Teesson M. *The measurement of consumer outcome in mental health: a report to the National Mental Health Information Strategy Committee.* Canberra, Australian Government Publishing Service, 1994.

26.   Ware J, Kosinski M, Keller SD. A 12-item short-form health survey: construction of scales and preliminary tests of reliability and validity. *Medical Care,* 1996, 34:220–233.

27.   The WHOQOL Group. Development of the World Health Organization WHOQOL-BREF quality of life assessment. *Psychological Medicine,* 1998, 28(3):551–558.

28.   World Health Organization. *ICF checklist.* Geneva, WHO, 2001.

29.   Chisholm D et al. Responsiveness of the World Health Organization Disability Assessment Schedule II (WHO DAS II) in a different cultural settings and health populaitons. *Submitted for publication,* 2009.

30.   Mokken RJ. *A theory and procedure of scale analysis.* The Hague, Mouton, 1971.

31.   Birnbaum A. Some latent trait models and their use in inferring an examinee's ability. In: Lord FM, Novick MR, eds. *Statistical theories of mental test scores.* Reading, MA, Addison Wesley, 1968.

32.   American Psychological Association. *Standards for educational and psychological tests.* Washington DC, APA, 1974.

33.   Chisolm T et al. The WHO-DAS II: psychometric properties in the measurement of functional health status in adults with acquired hearing loss. *Trends in Amplification,* 2005, 9:111–126.

34.   Üstün TB et al. WHO multi-country survey study on health and responsiveness 2000-2001. In: *Health systems performance assessment: debates, methods and empiricism.* Geneva, World Health Organization, 2003:761–796.

35.   Üstün TB et al. The world health surveys. In: Murray CJL, Evans DB, eds. *Health systems performance assessment: debates, methods and empiricism.* Geneva, World Health Organization, 2003.

36.   Kessler R, Ustün TB. *The WHO world mental health surveys: global perspectives on the epidemiology of mental disorders.* New York, Cambridge University Press, 2008.

37.   Baskett J et al. Functional disability in residents of Auckland rest homes. *New Zealand Medical Journal,* 1991, 104:200–202.

38.   Buist-Bouwman M et al. Psychometric properties of the World Health Organization Disability Assessment Schedule used in the European Study of the Epidemiology of Mental Disorders. *International Journal of Methods in Psychiatric Research,* 2008, 17(4):185–197.

39.   Scott K et al. Disability in Te Rau Hinengaro: the New Zealand mental health survey. *Australian and New Zealand Journal of Psychiatry,* 2006, 40(10):889–895.

40.   Reich J. DSM-III diagnoses in social security disability applicants referred for psychiatric evaluation. *Journal of Clinical Psychiatry,* 1986, 47(22):81–82.

41.   Alonso J et al. Disability and quality of life impact of mental disorders in Europe: results from the European Study of the Epidemiology of Mental Disorders (ESEMeD) project. *Acta Psychiatrica Scandinavica,* 2004, 109(Suppl 420):38–46.

42.   World Health Organization, United Nations Economic and Social Commission for Asia and the Pacific. *Training manual on disability statistics.* Bangkok, WHO and UNESCAP, 2008.

43.   O'Donovan M-A, Doyle A. *Measuring activity and participation of people with disabilities – an overview.* Dublin, Health Research Board, 2006.

44.   Gallagher P, Mulvany F. Levels of ability and functioning: using the WHODAS II in an Irish context. *Disability & Rehabilitation,* 2004, 26(9):506–517.

45.   Instituto Nacional de Estadísticas y Censos de Nicaragua (INEC). *Encuesta Nicaragüense para personas con discapacidad (ENIDS) 2003: Capítulo 2, Concepto y prevalencia de la discapacidad [Nicaraguan survey of persons with disability 2003: Chapter 2, Concepts and prevalence of disability].* Managua, INEC, 2003.

46.   Secretaria de Salud. Encuesta nacional de evaluación del disempeño, 2003 [National survey to evaluate ability, 2003]. In: *Programa nacional de salud 2007–2012 — Anexos.* México, Secretaria de Salud, 2007.

47.   Fondo Nacional de la Discapacidad (FONADIS). *Primer estudio nacional de la discapacidad en Chile (ENDISC 2004) [First national study of disability in Chile].* Santiago de Chile, FONADIS, 2005.

48.   Ministerio de Salud — Programa Nacional de Rehabilitación. *Certificación de la discapacidad en Nicaragua [Certification of disability in Nicaragua].* Managua, Ministerio de Salud — Programa Nacional de Rehabilitación, 2004.

49.   Ministerio de la Presidencia de la Republica de Panamá y Ministerio de Economía y Finanzas. *Estudio sobre la prevalencia y caracterización de la discapacidad en la República de Panamá [Study of the prevalence and character of disability in the Republic of Panama].* Panamá City, Ministerio de la Presidencia de la Republica de Panamá y Ministerio de Economía y Finanzas, 2006.

50.   United Nations Development Programme, World Health Organization, International Federation of Red Cross and Red Crescent Societies. *Tsunami recovery impact assessment and monitoring system (TRIAMS) — second regional TRIAMS workshop, Bangkok, 21–23 March 2007.* UNDP, WHO, IFRC, 2009.

51.   Federici S et al. World Health Organisation Disability Assessment Schedule II: contribution to the Italian validation. *Disability and rehabilitation,* 2009, 31(7):553–564.

52.   McGee R, Stanton W. Parents reports of disability among 13-year olds with DSM-III disorders. *The Journal of Child Psychology and Psychiatry and Allied Disciplines,* 1990, 31:793–801.

53.   Baron M et al. The clinimetric properties of the World Health Organization Disability Assessment Schedule II in early inflammatory arthritis. *Arthritis & Rheumatism,* 2008, 59(3):382–390.

54.   Schlote A et al. [Use of the WHODAS II with stroke patients and their relatives: reliability and inter-rater-reliability]. *Rehabilitation (Stuttg),* 2008, 47(1):31–38.

55.   Hudson M et al. Quality of life in systemic sclerosis: psychometric properties of the World Health Organization Disability Assessment Schedule II. *Arthritis & Rheumatism,* 2008, 59(2):270–278.

56.   McFarlane A. The international classification of impairments, disabilities and handicaps: its usefulness in classifying and understanding biopsychosocial phenomena. *Australian and New Zealand Journal of Psychiatry,* 1988, 22(1):31–42.

57.   Posl M, Cieza A, Stucki G. Psychometric properties of the WHODASII in rehabilitation patients. *Quality of Life Research,* 2007, 16(9):1521–1531.

58.   Soberg H et al. Long-term multidimensional functional consequences of severe multiple injuries two years after trauma: a prospective longitudinal cohort study. *Journal of Trauma,* 2007, 62(2):461–470.

59.   Bryan S, Parkin D, Donaldson C. Chiropody and the QALY: a case study in assigning categories of disability and distress to patients. *Health Policy,* 1991, 18:169–185.

60.   Kim J et al. Physical health, depression and cognitive function as correlates of disability in an older Korean population. *International Journal of Geriatric Psychiatry,* 2005, 20(2):160–167.

61.   Chopra P, Couper J, Herrman H. The assessment of patients with long-term psychotic disorders: application of the WHO Disability Assessment Schedule II. *Australian and New Zealand Journal of Psychiatry,* 2004, 38(9):753–759.

62.   Ertugrul A, Ulug B. Perception of stigma among patients with schizophrenia. *Social Psychiatry and Psychiatric Epidemiology,* 2004, 39(1):73–77.

63.   Annicchiarico R et al. Qualitative profiles of disability. *Journal of Rehabilitation Research and Development,* 2004, 41(6A):835–846.

64.   McKibbin C, Patterson T, Jeste D. Assessing disability in older patients with schizophrenia: results from the WHODAS-II. *Journal of Nervous and Mental Disease,* 2004, 192:405–413.

65.   Norton J et al. Psychiatric morbidity, disability and service use amongst primary care attenders in France. *European Psychiatry,* 2004, 19:164–167.

66.   The Mental Health and General Practice Investigation (MaGPIe) Research Group. General practitioner recognition of mental illness in the absence of a 'gold standard'. *Australian and New Zealand Journal of Psychiatry,* 2004, 38:789–794.

67.   Kemmler G et al. Quality of life of HIV-infected patients: psychometric properties and validation of the German version of the MQOL-HIV. *Quality of Life Research,* 2003, 12:1037–1050.

68.   Edwards G, Arif A, Hodgson R. Nomenclature and classification of drug- and alcohol-related problems: a WHO memorandum. *Bulletin of the World Health Organization,* 1981, 59:225–242.

69.   Chwastiak L, Von KM. Disability in depression and back pain: evaluation of the World Health Organization Disability Assessment Schedule (WHO DAS II) in a primary care setting. *Journal of Clinical Epidemiology,* 2003, 56(6):507–514.

70.   Chwastiak L, Von Korff M. Disability in depression and back pain: responsiveness to change of the WHO Disability Assessment Schedule (WHO DAS II) in a primary care setting. *Journal of Clinical Epidemiology,* 2003, 56:507–514.

71.   Van Tubergen A et al. Assessment of disability with the World Health Organization Disability Assessment Schedule II in patients with ankylosing spondylitis. *Annals of the Rheumatic Diseases,* 2003, 62:140–145.

72.   Olivera Roulet G. *La aplicación de la CIF en la Argentina desde el ano 2003 [The application of CIF in Argentina since 2003].* Buenos Aires, Ministerio de Salud – Servicio Nacional de Rehabilitación, 2007.

73.   Wing J, Sartorius N, Üstün TB. *Diagnosis and clinical measurement in psychiatry, a reference manual for the SCAN system.* Cambridge, Cambridge University Press, 1995.

74.   Üstün TB et al. Multiple-informant ranking of the disabling effects of different health conditions in 14 countries. WHO/NIH Joint Project CAR Study Group. *Lancet,* 1999, 354(9173):111–115.

75.   Lord F, Novick M. *Statistical theories of mental test scores.* Reading, MA, Addison Wesley, 1968.

76.   Rasch G. *Probabilistic models for some intelligence and attainment tests. 2nd edition.* Chicago, University of Chicago Press, 1980.

77.   Ford B. An overview of hot-deck procedures. In: Madow W, Olkin I, Rubin D, eds. *Incomplete data in sample surveys.* Academic Press, New York, 1983:185–207.

78.   Rubin D. *Multiple imputation for nonresponse in surveys.* New York, John Wiley & Sons, 1987.

Part 3

WHODAS 2.0 VERSIONS

This section contains the seven paper-based versions of WHODAS 2.0:

- three 36-item versions:
  - interview-administered
  - self-administered
  - proxy-administered
- three 12-item versions:
  - interview-administered
  - self-administered
  - proxy-administered
- one 12+24-item version:
  - interview-administered.

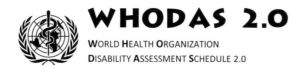

WHODAS 2.0

WORLD **H**EALTH **O**RGANIZATION
DISABILITY **A**SSESSMENT **S**CHEDULE 2.0

36-item version, interviewer-administered

Introduction

This instrument was developed by the WHO *Classification, Terminology and Standards* team, within the framework of the WHO/National Institutes of Health (NIH) Joint Project on Assessment and Classification of Disability.

Before using this instrument, interviewers must be trained using the manual *Measuring Health and Disability: Manual for WHO Disability Assessment Schedule – WHODAS 2.0* (WHO 2010), which includes an interview guide and other training material.

The versions of the interview available are as follows:

- 36-item – Interviewer-administered[a]
- 36-item – Self-administered
- 36-item – Proxy-administered[b]
- 12-item – Interviewer-administered[c]
- 12-item – Self-administered
- 12-item – Proxy-administered
- 12+24-item – Interviewer-administered

  [a] A computerized version of the interview (*iShell*) is available for computer-assisted interviews or for data entry
  [b] Relatives, friends or caretakers
  [c] The 12-item version explains 81% of the variance of the more detailed 36-item version

For more details of the versions please refer to the WHODAS 2.0 manual *Measuring Health and Disability: Manual for WHO Disability Assessment Schedule – WHODAS 2.0* (WHO 2010).

Permission to translate this instrument into any language should be obtained from WHO, and all translations should be prepared according to the WHO translation guidelines, as detailed in the accompanying manual.

For additional information, please visit www.who.int/whodas or contact:

Dr T Bedirhan Üstün
Classification, Terminology and Standards
Health Statistics and Informatics
World Health Organization (WHO)
1211 Geneva 27
Switzerland

Tel: + 41 22 791 3609
E-mail:ustunb@who.int

WHODAS 2.0

WORLD HEALTH ORGANIZATION
DISABILITY ASSESSMENT SCHEDULE 2.0

This questionnaire contains the interviewer-administered 36-item version of WHODAS 2.0.

Instructions to the interviewer are written in bold and italics – do not read these aloud.

Text for the respondent to hear is written in

standard print in blue.

Read this text aloud.

Section 1   Face sheet

Complete items F1–F5 before starting each interview				
F1	Respondent identity number			
F2	Interviewer identity number			
F3	Assessment time point (1, 2, etc.)			
F4	Interview date	——— day	——— month	——— year
F5	Living situation at time of interview (circle only one)	Independent in community		1
		Assisted living		2
		Hospitalized		3

Section 2   Demographic and background information

This interview has been developed by the World Health Organization (WHO) to better understand the difficulties people may have due to their health conditions. The information that you provide in this interview is confidential and will be used only for research. The interview will take 15–20 minutes to complete.

For respondents from the general population (not the clinical population) say:

Even if you are healthy and have no difficulties, I need to ask all of the questions so that the survey is complete.

I will start with some background questions.

A1	**Record sex as observed**	Female	1
		Male	2
A2	How old are you now?	_____ years	
A3	How many years in all did you spend <u>studying in school</u>, college or university?	_____ years	
A4	What is your <u>current marital status</u>? **(Select the single best option)**	Never married	1
		Currently married	2
		Separated	3
		Divorced	4
		Widowed	5
		Cohabiting	6
A5	Which describes your <u>main work status</u> best? **(Select the single best option)**	Paid work	1
		Self employed, such as own your business or farming	2
		Non-paid work, such as volunteer or charity	3
		Student	4
		Keeping house/ homemaker	5
		Retired	6
		Unemployed (health reasons)	7
		Unemployed (other reasons)	8
		Other (specify)_____ _____	9

Section 3   Preamble

Say to respondent:

The interview is about difficulties people have because of health conditions.

Hand flashcard #1 to respondent and say:

By health condition I mean diseases or illnesses, or other health problems that may be short or long lasting; injuries; mental or emotional problems; and problems with alcohol or drugs.

Remember to keep all of your health problems in mind as you answer the questions. When I ask you about difficulties in doing an activity think about …

Point to flashcard #1 and explain that "difficulty with an activity" means:

*   Increased effort
*   Discomfort or pain
*   Slowness
*   Changes in the way you do the activity.

Say to respondent:

When answering, I'd like you to think back over the past 30 days. I would also like you to answer these questions thinking about how much difficulty you have had, on average, over the past 30 days, while doing the activity as you usually do it.

Hand flashcard #2 to respondent and say:

Use this scale when responding.

Read the scale aloud:

None, mild, moderate, severe, extreme or cannot do.

Ensure that the respondent can easily see flashcards #1 and #2 throughout the interview

Section 4 Domain reviews

Domain 1 Cognition

I am now going to ask some questions about <u>understanding and communicating.</u>

Show flashcards #1 and #2 to respondent

In the past 30 days, how much difficulty did you have in:		None	Mild	Moderate	Severe	Extreme or cannot do
D1.1	<u>Concentrating</u> on doing something for <u>ten minutes</u>?	1	2	3	4	5
D1.2	<u>Remembering</u> to do <u>important things</u>?	1	2	3	4	5
D1.3	<u>Analysing and finding solutions to problems</u> in day-to-day life?	1	2	3	4	5
D1.4	<u>Learning</u> a <u>new task</u>, for example, learning how to get to a new place?	1	2	3	4	5
D1.5	<u>Generally understanding</u> what people say?	1	2	3	4	5
D1.6	<u>Starting and maintaining a conversation</u>?	1	2	3	4	5

Domain 2 Mobility

I am now going to ask you about difficulties in <u>getting around</u>.

Show flashcards #1 and #2

In the past 30 days, how much difficulty did you have in:		None	Mild	Moderate	Severe	Extreme or cannot do
D2.1	<u>Standing</u> for <u>long periods</u> such as <u>30 minutes</u>?	1	2	3	4	5
D2.2	<u>Standing up</u> from sitting down?	1	2	3	4	5
D2.3	<u>Moving</u> around <u>inside your home</u>?	1	2	3	4	5
D2.4	<u>Getting out</u> of your <u>home</u>?	1	2	3	4	5
D2.5	<u>Walking a long distance</u> such as a <u>kilometre</u> [or equivalent]?	1	2	3	4	5

Please continue to next page...

Domain 3   Self-care

I am now going to ask you about difficulties in <u>taking care of yourself</u>.

Show flashcards #1 and #2

In the past <u>30 days</u>, how much <u>difficulty</u> did you have in:		None	Mild	Moderate	Severe	Extreme or cannot do
D3.1	<u>Washing</u> your <u>whole body</u>?	1	2	3	4	5
D3.2	Getting <u>dressed</u>?	1	2	3	4	5
D3.3	<u>Eating</u>?	1	2	3	4	5
D3.4	Staying <u>by yourself</u> for a <u>few days</u>?	1	2	3	4	5

Domain 4   Getting along with people

I am now going to ask you about difficulties in <u>getting along with people</u>. Please remember that I am asking only about difficulties that are due to health problems. By this I mean diseases or illnesses, injuries, mental or emotional problems and problems with alcohol or drugs.

Show flashcards #1 and #2

In the past 30 days, how much difficulty did you have in:		None	Mild	Moderate	Severe	Extreme or cannot do
D4.1	<u>Dealing with people you do not know</u>?	1	2	3	4	5
D4.2	<u>Maintaining a friendship</u>?	1	2	3	4	5
D4.3	<u>Getting along</u> with people who are <u>close</u> to you?	1	2	3	4	5
D4.4	<u>Making new friends</u>?	1	2	3	4	5
D4.5	<u>Sexual activities</u>?	1	2	3	4	5

Please continue to next page...

Domain 5   Life activities

5(1)   Household activities

I am now going to ask you about activities involved in maintaining your household, and in caring for the people who you live with or are close to. These activities include cooking, cleaning, shopping, caring for others and caring for your belongings.

Show flashcards #1 and #2

Because of your health condition, in the past 30 days, how much difficulty did you have in:		None	Mild	Moderate	Severe	Extreme or cannot do
D5.1	Taking care of your <u>household responsibilities</u>?	1	2	3	4	5
D5.2	Doing your most important household tasks <u>well</u>?	1	2	3	4	5
D5.3	Getting all the household work <u>done</u> that you needed to do?	1	2	3	4	5
D5.4	Getting your household work done as <u>quickly</u> as needed?	1	2	3	4	5

If any of the responses to D5.2–D5.5 are rated greater than none (coded as "1"), ask:

D5.01	In the past 30 days, on how many days did you reduce or completely miss <u>household work</u> because of your health condition?	*Record number of days* ____

If respondent works (paid, non-paid, self-employed) or goes to school, complete questions D5.5–D5.10 on the next page. Otherwise, skip to D6.1 on the following page.

5(2)   Work or school activities

Now I will ask some questions about your work or school activities.

Show flashcards #1 and #2

Because of your health condition, in the past 30 days how much difficulty did you have in:		None	Mild	Moderate	Severe	Extreme or cannot do
D5.5	Your day-to-day work/school?	1	2	3	4	5
D5.6	Doing your most important work/school tasks well?	1	2	3	4	5
D5.7	Getting all the work done that you need to do?	1	2	3	4	5
D5.8	Getting your work done as quickly as needed?	1	2	3	4	5
D5.9	Have you had to work at a lower level because of a health condition?				No	1
					Yes	2
D5.10	Did you earn less money as the result of a health condition?				No	1
					Yes	2

If any of D5.5–D5.8 are rated greater than none (coded as "1"), ask:

D5.02	In the past 30 days, on how many days did you miss work for half a day or more because of your health condition?	*Record number of days* ____

Please continue to next page...

Domain 6   Participation

Now, I am going to ask you about <u>your participation in society</u> and the <u>impact of your health problems</u> on <u>you and your family</u>. Some of these questions may involve problems that go beyond the past 30 days, however in answering, please focus on the past 30 days. Again, I remind you to answer these questions while thinking about health problems: physical, mental or emotional, alcohol or drug related.

Show flashcards #1 and #2

In the past 30 days:		None	Mild	Moderate	Severe	Extreme or cannot do
D6.1	How much of a problem did you have <u>joining in community activities</u> (for example, festivities, religious or other activities) in the same way as anyone else can?	1	2	3	4	5
D6.2	How much of a problem did you have because of <u>barriers or hindrances</u> in the world around you?	1	2	3	4	5
D6.3	How much of a problem did you have <u>living with dignity</u> because of the attitudes and actions of others?	1	2	3	4	5
D6.4	How much <u>time</u> did <u>you</u> spend on your health condition or its consequences?	1	2	3	4	5
D6.5	How much have <u>you</u> been <u>emotionally affected</u> by your health condition?	1	2	3	4	5
D6.6	How much has your health been a <u>drain on the financial resources</u> of you or your family?	1	2	3	4	5
D6.7	How much of a problem did your <u>family</u> have because of your health problems?	1	2	3	4	5
D6.8	How much of a problem did you have in doing things <u>by yourself</u> for <u>relaxation or pleasure</u>?	1	2	3	4	5

H1	Overall, in the past 30 days, <u>how many days</u> were these difficulties present?	*Record number of days* ____
H2	In the past 30 days, for how many days were you <u>totally unable</u> to carry out your usual activities or work because of any health condition?	*Record number of days* ____
H3	In the past 30 days, not counting the days that you were totally unable, for how many days did you <u>cut back</u> or <u>reduce</u> your usual activities or work because of any health condition?	*Record number of days* ____

This concludes the interview. Thank you for participating.

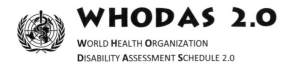

WHODAS 2.0
WORLD HEALTH ORGANIZATION
DISABILITY ASSESSMENT SCHEDULE 2.0

Health conditions:

- **Diseases, illnesses or other health problems**
- **Injuries**
- **Mental or emotional problems**
- **Problems with alcohol**
- **Problems with drugs**

Having difficulty with an activity means:

- **Increased effort**
- **Discomfort or pain**
- **Slowness**
- **Changes in the way you do the activity**

Think about the past 30 days only.

WHODAS 2.0

WORLD HEALTH ORGANIZATION
DISABILITY ASSESSMENT SCHEDULE 2.0

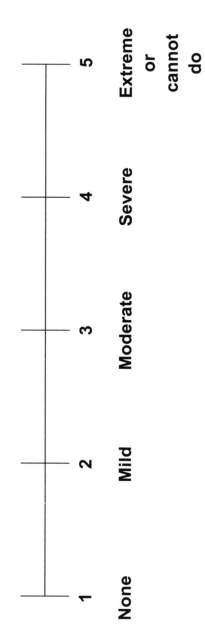

1	2	3	4	5
None	Mild	Moderate	Severe	Extreme or cannot do

WHODAS 2.0

WORLD HEALTH ORGANIZATION
DISABILITY ASSESSMENT SCHEDULE 2.0

36-item version, self-administered

This questionnaire asks about <u>difficulties due to health conditions</u>. Health conditions include diseases or illnesses, other health problems that may be short or long lasting, injuries, mental or emotional problems, and problems with alcohol or drugs.

Think back over the <u>past 30 days</u> and answer these questions, thinking about how much difficulty you had doing the following activities. For each question, please circle only <u>one</u> response.

In the past <u>30 days</u>, how much <u>difficulty</u> did you have in:						
Understanding and communicating						
D1.1	<u>Concentrating</u> on doing something for <u>ten minutes</u>?	None	Mild	Moderate	Severe	Extreme or cannot do
D1.2	<u>Remembering</u> to do <u>important things</u>?	None	Mild	Moderate	Severe	Extreme or cannot do
D1.3	<u>Analysing and finding solutions to problems</u> in day-to-day life?	None	Mild	Moderate	Severe	Extreme or cannot do
D1.4	<u>Learning</u> a <u>new task</u>, for example, learning how to get to a new place?	None	Mild	Moderate	Severe	Extreme or cannot do
D1.5	<u>Generally understanding</u> what people say?	None	Mild	Moderate	Severe	Extreme or cannot do
D1.6	<u>Starting and maintaining</u> a <u>conversation</u>?	None	Mild	Moderate	Severe	Extreme or cannot do
Getting around						
D2.1	<u>Standing</u> for <u>long periods</u> such as <u>30 minutes</u>?	None	Mild	Moderate	Severe	Extreme or cannot do
D2.2	<u>Standing up</u> from sitting down?	None	Mild	Moderate	Severe	Extreme or cannot do
D2.3	<u>Moving</u> around <u>inside your home</u>?	None	Mild	Moderate	Severe	Extreme or cannot do
D2.4	<u>Getting out</u> of your <u>home</u>?	None	Mild	Moderate	Severe	Extreme or cannot do
D2.5	<u>Walking a long distance</u> such as a <u>kilometre</u> [or equivalent]?	None	Mild	Moderate	Severe	Extreme or cannot do

Please continue to next page …

In the past <u>30 days</u>, how much <u>difficulty</u> did you have in:						
Self-care						
D3.1	<u>Washing</u> your <u>whole body</u>?	None	Mild	Moderate	Severe	Extreme or cannot do
D3.2	Getting <u>dressed</u>?	None	Mild	Moderate	Severe	Extreme or cannot do
D3.3	<u>Eating</u>?	None	Mild	Moderate	Severe	Extreme or cannot do
D3.4	Staying <u>by yourself</u> for a <u>few days</u>?	None	Mild	Moderate	Severe	Extreme or cannot do
Getting along with people						
D4.1	<u>Dealing</u> with people <u>you do not know</u>?	None	Mild	Moderate	Severe	Extreme or cannot do
D4.2	<u>Maintaining a friendship</u>?	None	Mild	Moderate	Severe	Extreme or cannot do
D4.3	<u>Getting along</u> with people who are <u>close</u> to you?	None	Mild	Moderate	Severe	Extreme or cannot do
D4.4	<u>Making new friends</u>?	None	Mild	Moderate	Severe	Extreme or cannot do
D4.5	<u>Sexual activities</u>?	None	Mild	Moderate	Severe	Extreme or cannot do
Life activities						
D5.1	Taking care of your <u>household responsibilities</u>?	None	Mild	Moderate	Severe	Extreme or cannot do
D5.2	Doing most important household tasks <u>well</u>?	None	Mild	Moderate	Severe	Extreme or cannot do
D5.3	Getting all the household work <u>done</u> that you needed to do?	None	Mild	Moderate	Severe	Extreme or cannot do
D5.4	Getting your household work done as <u>quickly</u> as needed?	None	Mild	Moderate	Severe	Extreme or cannot do

Please continue to next page …

If you work (paid, non-paid, self-employed) or go to school, complete questions D5.5–D5.8, below. Otherwise, skip to D6.1.

Because of your health condition, in the past <u>30 days</u>, how much <u>difficulty</u> did you have in:						
D5.5	Your day-to-day <u>work/school</u>?	None	Mild	Moderate	Severe	Extreme or cannot do
D5.6	Doing your most important work/school tasks <u>well</u>?	None	Mild	Moderate	Severe	Extreme or cannot do
D5.7	Getting all the work <u>done</u> that you need to do?	None	Mild	Moderate	Severe	Extreme or cannot do
D5.8	Getting your work done as <u>quickly</u> as needed?	None	Mild	Moderate	Severe	Extreme or cannot do

Participation in society						
In the past <u>30 days</u>:						
D6.1	How much of a problem did you have in <u>joining in community activities</u> (for example, festivities, religious or other activities) in the same way as anyone else can?	None	Mild	Moderate	Severe	Extreme or cannot do
D6.2	How much of a problem did you have because of <u>barriers or hindrances</u> in the world around you?	None	Mild	Moderate	Severe	Extreme or cannot do
D6.3	How much of a problem did you have <u>living with dignity</u> because of the attitudes and actions of others?	None	Mild	Moderate	Severe	Extreme or cannot do
D6.4	How much <u>time</u> did <u>you</u> spend on your health condition, or its consequences?	None	Mild	Moderate	Severe	Extreme or cannot do
D6.5	How much have <u>you</u> been <u>emotionally affected</u> by your health condition?	None	Mild	Moderate	Severe	Extreme or cannot do
D6.6	How much has your health been a <u>drain on the financial resources</u> of you or your family?	None	Mild	Moderate	Severe	Extreme or cannot do
D6.7	How much of a problem did your <u>family</u> have because of your health problems?	None	Mild	Moderate	Severe	Extreme or cannot do
D6.8	How much of a problem did you have in doing things <u>by yourself</u> for <u>relaxation or pleasure</u>?	None	Mild	Moderate	Severe	Extreme or cannot do

Please continue to next page …

H1	Overall, in the past 30 days, <u>how many days</u> were these difficulties present?	*Record number of days* ____
H2	In the past 30 days, for how many days were you <u>totally unable</u> to carry out your usual activities or work because of any health condition?	*Record number of days* ____
H3	In the past 30 days, not counting the days that you were totally unable, for how many days did you <u>cut back</u> or <u>reduce</u> your usual activities or work because of any health condition?	*Record number of days* ____

This completes the questionnaire. Thank you.

WHODAS 2.0

WORLD **H**EALTH **O**RGANIZATION
DISABILITY **A**SSESSMENT **S**CHEDULE 2.0

36-item version, proxy-administered

This questionnaire asks about <u>difficulties due to health conditions</u> experienced by the person about whom you are responding in your role as friend, relative or carer. Health conditions include diseases or illnesses, other health problems that may be short or long lasting, injuries, mental or emotional problems, and problems with alcohol or drugs.

Think back over the <u>past 30 days</u> and, to the best of your knowledge, answer these questions thinking about how much difficulty your <u>friend, relative or carer</u> had while doing the following activities. (Note: the questionnaire uses the term "relative" to mean "friend", "relative" or "carer".) For each question, please circle only <u>one</u> response.

H4[a]	I am the _____ (choose one) of this person.	1 =	husband or wife	5 =	other relative
		2 =	parent	6 =	friend
		3 =	son or daughter	7 =	professional carer
		4 =	brother or sister	8 =	other (specify) _____

[a] Questions H1–H3 appear at the end of the questionnaire.

Please continue to next page …

In the past 30 days, <u>how much difficulty</u> did your relative have in:						
Understanding and communicating						
D1.1	Concentrating on doing something for ten minutes?	None	Mild	Moderate	Severe	Extreme or cannot do
D1.2	Remembering to do important things?	None	Mild	Moderate	Severe	Extreme or cannot do
D1.3	Analysing and finding solutions to problems in day-to-day life?	None	Mild	Moderate	Severe	Extreme or cannot do
D1.4	Learning a new task, for example, learning how to get to a new place?	None	Mild	Moderate	Severe	Extreme or cannot do
D1.5	Generally understanding what people say?	None	Mild	Moderate	Severe	Extreme or cannot do
D1.6	Starting and maintaining a conversation?	None	Mild	Moderate	Severe	Extreme or cannot do
Getting around						
D2.1	Standing for long periods such as 30 minutes?	None	Mild	Moderate	Severe	Extreme or cannot do
D2.2	Standing up from sitting down?	None	Mild	Moderate	Severe	Extreme or cannot do
D2.3	Moving around inside their home?	None	Mild	Moderate	Severe	Extreme or cannot do
D2.4	Getting out of their home?	None	Mild	Moderate	Severe	Extreme or cannot do
D2.5	Walking a long distance such as a kilometre [or equivalent]?	None	Mild	Moderate	Severe	Extreme or cannot do

Please continue to next page ...

Because of their health condition, in the past 30 days, <u>how much difficulty</u> did your relative have in:

Self-care

D3.1	<u>Washing</u> his or her <u>whole body</u>?	None	Mild	Moderate	Severe	Extreme or cannot do
D3.2	Getting <u>dressed?</u>	None	Mild	Moderate	Severe	Extreme or cannot do
D3.3	<u>Eating</u>?	None	Mild	Moderate	Severe	Extreme or cannot do
D3.4	Staying <u>by himself or herself</u> for a <u>few days</u>?	None	Mild	Moderate	Severe	Extreme or cannot do

Getting along with people

D4.1	<u>Dealing with people he or she does not know</u>?	None	Mild	Moderate	Severe	Extreme or cannot do
D4.2	<u>Maintaining a friendship</u>?	None	Mild	Moderate	Severe	Extreme or cannot do
D4.3	<u>Getting along</u> with people who are <u>close</u> to him or her?	None	Mild	Moderate	Severe	Extreme or cannot do
D4.4	<u>Making new friends</u>?	None	Mild	Moderate	Severe	Extreme or cannot do
D4.5	<u>Sexual</u> activities?	None	Mild	Moderate	Severe	Extreme or cannot do

Life activities

D5.1	Taking care of his or her <u>household responsibilities</u>?	None	Mild	Moderate	Severe	Extreme or cannot do
D5.2	Doing his or her most important household tasks <u>well</u>?	None	Mild	Moderate	Severe	Extreme or cannot do
D5.3	Getting all the household work <u>done</u> that is needed?	None	Mild	Moderate	Severe	Extreme or cannot do
D5.4	Getting the household work done as <u>quickly</u> as needed?	None	Mild	Moderate	Severe	Extreme or cannot do

If your relative works (paid, non-paid, self-employed) or goes to school, complete questions D5.5–D5.8, below. Otherwise, skip to D6.1 near the top of the following page.

In the past <u>30 days,</u> <u>how much difficulty</u> did your relative have in:						
D5.5	His or her day-to-day <u>work/school</u>?	None	Mild	Moderate	Severe	Extreme or cannot do
D5.6	Doing his or her most important work/ school tasks <u>well</u>?	None	Mild	Moderate	Severe	Extreme or cannot do
D5.7	Getting all the work <u>done</u> that is needed?	None	Mild	Moderate	Severe	Extreme or cannot do
D5.8	Getting the work done as <u>quickly</u> as needed?	None	Mild	Moderate	Severe	Extreme or cannot do

Participation in society in the <u>past 30 days</u>						
D6.1	How much of a problem did <u>your relative</u> have in <u>joining in community activities</u> (for example, festivities, religious or other activities) in the same way as anyone else can?	None	Mild	Moderate	Severe	Extreme or cannot do
D6.2	How much of a problem did your relative have because of <u>barriers or hindrances</u> in the world around him or her?	None	Mild	Moderate	Severe	Extreme or cannot do
D6.3	How much of a problem did your relative have <u>living with dignity</u> because of the attitudes and actions of others?	None	Mild	Moderate	Severe	Extreme or cannot do
D6.4	How much <u>time</u> did <u>your relative</u> spend on his or her health condition, or its consequences?	None	Mild	Moderate	Severe	Extreme or cannot do
D6.5	How much has <u>your relative</u> been <u>emotionally affected</u> by his or her health condition?	None	Mild	Moderate	Severe	Extreme or cannot do
D6.6	How much has his or her health been a <u>drain on his or her financial resources</u> or on the financial resources of other relatives?	None	Mild	Moderate	Severe	Extreme or cannot do
D6.7	How much of a problem did <u>you</u> or the <u>rest of his or her family</u> have because of his or her health problems?	None	Mild	Moderate	Severe	Extreme or cannot do
D6.8	How much of a problem did your relative have in doing things <u>by himself or herself</u> for <u>relaxation or pleasure</u>?	None	Mild	Moderate	Severe	Extreme or cannot do

Please continue to next page …

H1	Overall, in the past 30 days, <u>how many days</u> were these difficulties present?	*Record number of days* ____
H2	In the past 30 days, for how many days was your relative <u>totally unable</u> to carry out his or her usual activities or work because of any health condition?	*Record number of days* ____
H3	In the past 30 days, not counting the days that your relative was totally unable, for how many days did your relative <u>cut back</u> or <u>reduce</u> his or her usual activities or work because of any health condition?	*Record number of days* ____

This completes the questionnaire. Thank you for participating.

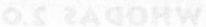

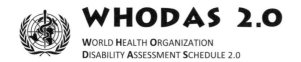

WHODAS 2.0

WORLD **H**EALTH **O**RGANIZATION
DISABILITY **A**SSESSMENT **S**CHEDULE 2.0

12-item version, interviewer-administered

Introduction

This instrument was developed by the WHO *Classification, Terminology and Standards* team, within the framework of the WHO/National Institutes of Health (NIH) Joint Project on Assessment and Classification of Disability.

Before using this instrument, interviewers must be trained using the manual *Measuring Health and Disability: Manual for WHO Disability Assessment Schedule – WHODAS 2.0* (WHO, 2010), which includes an interview guide and other training material.

The versions of the interview available are as follows:

- 36-item – Interviewer-administered[a]
- 36-item – Self-administered
- 36-item – Proxy-administered[b]
- 12-item – Interviewer-administered[c]
- 12-item – Self-administered
- 12-item – Proxy-administered
- 12+24-item – Interviewer-administered

[a] A computerized version of the interview (*iShell*) is available for computer-assisted interviews or for data entry
[b] Relatives, friends or caretakers
[c] The 12-item version explains 81% of the variance of the more detailed 36-item version

For more details of the versions please refer to the WHODAS 2.0 manual *Measuring Health and Disability: Manual for WHO Disability Assessment Schedule – WHODAS 2.0* (WHO, 2010).

Permission to translate this instrument into any language should be obtained from WHO, and all translations should be prepared according to the WHO translation guidelines, as detailed in the accompanying manual.

For additional information, please visit www.who.int/whodas or contact:

Dr T Bedirhan Üstün
Classification, Terminology and Standards
Health Statistics and Informatics
World Health Organization (WHO)
1211 Geneva 27
Switzerland

Tel: + 41 22 791 3609
E-mail:ustunb@who.int

This questionnaire contains the interviewer-administered, 12-item version of WHODAS 2.0.

Instructions to the interviewer are written in bold and italics – do not read these aloud

Text for the respondent to hear is written in

standard print in blue.

Read this text aloud

Section 1   Face sheet

Complete items F1–F5 before starting each interview				
F1	Respondent identity number			
F2	Interviewer identity number			
F3	Assessment time point (1, 2, etc)			
F4	Interview date	_____ day	_____ month	_____ year
F5	Living situation at time of interview (circle only one)	Independent in community		1
		Assisted living		2
		Hospitalized		3

Please continue to next page ...

Section 2   Demographic and background information

This interview has been developed by the World Health Organization (WHO) to better understand the difficulties people may have due to their health conditions. The information that you provide in this interview is confidential and will be used only for research. The interview will take 5–10 minutes to complete.

For respondents from the general population (not the clinical population) say:

Even if you are healthy and have no difficulties, I need to ask all of the questions so that the survey is complete.

I will start with some background questions.

A1	**Record sex as observed**	Female	1
		Male	2
A2	How old are you now?	_____ years	
A3	How many years in all did you spend studying in school, college or university?	_____ years	
A4	What is your current marital status? **(Select the single best option)**	Never married	1
		Currently married	2
		Separated	3
		Divorced	4
		Widowed	5
		Cohabiting	6
A5	Which describes your main work status best? **(Select the single best option)**	Paid work	1
		Self-employed, such as own your business or farming	2
		Non-paid work, such as volunteer or charity	3
		Student	4
		Keeping house/ homemaker	5
		Retired	6
		Unemployed (health reasons)	7
		Unemployed (other reasons)	8
		Other (specify)_____ _____	9

Please continue to next page...

Section 3   Preamble

Say to respondent:

The interview is about difficulties people have because of health conditions.

Hand flashcard #1 to respondent

By health condition I mean diseases or illnesses, or other health problems that may be short or long lasting; injuries; mental or emotional problems; and problems with alcohol or drugs.

Remember to keep all of your health problems in mind as you answer the questions. When I ask you about difficulties in doing an activity think about...

Point to flashcard #1

- Increased effort
- Discomfort or pain
- Slowness
- Changes in the way you do the activity.

When answering, I'd like you to think back over the past 30 days. I would also like you to answer these questions thinking about how much difficulty you have had, on average, over the past 30 days, while doing the activity as you <u>usually</u> do it.

Hand flashcard #2 to respondent

Use this scale when responding.

Read scale aloud:

None, mild, moderate, severe, extreme or cannot do.

Ensure that the respondent can easily see flashcards #1 and #2 throughout the interview

Please continue to next page...

Section 4   Core questions

Show flashcard #2

In the past 30 days, how much difficulty did you have in:		None	Mild	Moderate	Severe	Extreme or cannot do
S1	Standing for long periods such as 30 minutes?	1	2	3	4	5
S2	Taking care of your household responsibilities?	1	2	3	4	5
S3	Learning a new task, for example, learning how to get to a new place?	1	2	3	4	5
S4	How much of a problem did you have joining in community activities (for example, festivities, religious or other activities) in the same way as anyone else can?	1	2	3	4	5
S5	How much have you been emotionally affected by your health problems?	1	2	3	4	5

In the past 30 days, how much difficulty did you have in:		None	Mild	Moderate	Severe	Extreme or cannot do
S6	Concentrating on doing something for ten minutes?	1	2	3	4	5
S7	Walking a long distance such as a kilometre [or equivalent]?	1	2	3	4	5
S8	Washing your whole body?	1	2	3	4	5
S9	Getting dressed?	1	2	3	4	5
S10	Dealing with people you do not know?	1	2	3	4	5
S11	Maintaining a friendship?	1	2	3	4	5
S12	Your day-to-day work/school?	1	2	3	4	5

H1	Overall, in the past 30 days, how many days were these difficulties present?	*Record number of days* ____
H2	In the past 30 days, for how many days were you totally unable to carry out your usual activities or work because of any health condition?	*Record number of days* ____
H3	In the past 30 days, not counting the days that you were totally unable, for how many days did you cut back or reduce your usual activities or work because of any health condition?	*Record number of days* ____

This concludes our interview. Thank you for participating.

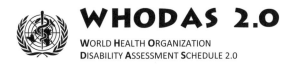

WHODAS 2.0
WORLD **H**EALTH **O**RGANIZATION
DISABILITY **A**SSESSMENT **S**CHEDULE 2.0

Health conditions:

- **Diseases, illnesses or other health problems**
- **Injuries**
- **Mental or emotional problems**
- **Problems with alcohol**
- **Problems with drugs**

Having difficulty with an activity means:

- **Increased effort**
- **Discomfort or pain**
- **Slowness**
- **Changes in the way you do the activity**

Think about the past 30 days only.

WHODAS 2.0

WORLD HEALTH ORGANIZATION
DISABILITY ASSESSMENT SCHEDULE 2.0

Flashcard 2

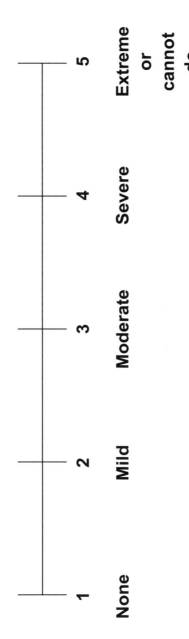

1	2	3	4	5
None	Mild	Moderate	Severe	Extreme or cannot do

WHODAS 2.0

WORLD HEALTH ORGANIZATION
DISABILITY ASSESSMENT SCHEDULE 2.0

12-item version, self-administered

This questionnaire asks about <u>difficulties due to health conditions</u>. Health conditions include diseases or illnesses, other health problems that may be short or long lasting, injuries, mental or emotional problems, and problems with alcohol or drugs.

Think back over the <u>past 30 days</u> and answer these questions, thinking about how much difficulty you had doing the following activities. For each question, please circle only <u>one</u> response.

In the past 30 days, how much difficulty did you have in:						
S1	<u>Standing</u> for <u>long periods</u> such as <u>30 minutes</u>?	None	Mild	Moderate	Severe	Extreme or cannot do
S2	Taking care of your <u>household responsibilities</u>?	None	Mild	Moderate	Severe	Extreme or cannot do
S3	<u>Learning</u> a <u>new task</u>, for example, learning how to get to a new place?	None	Mild	Moderate	Severe	Extreme or cannot do
S4	How much of a problem did you have <u>joining in community activities</u> (for example, festivities, religious or other activities) in the same way as anyone else can?	None	Mild	Moderate	Severe	Extreme or cannot do
S5	How much have <u>you</u> been <u>emotionally affected</u> by your health problems?	None	Mild	Moderate	Severe	Extreme or cannot do

Please continue to next page...

In the past 30 days, how much difficulty did you have in:						
S6	Concentrating on doing something for ten minutes?	None	Mild	Moderate	Severe	Extreme or cannot do
S7	Walking a long distance such as a kilometre [or equivalent]?	None	Mild	Moderate	Severe	Extreme or cannot do
S8	Washing your whole body?	None	Mild	Moderate	Severe	Extreme or cannot do
S9	Getting dressed?	None	Mild	Moderate	Severe	Extreme or cannot do
S10	Dealing with people you do not know?	None	Mild	Moderate	Severe	Extreme or cannot do
S11	Maintaining a friendship?	None	Mild	Moderate	Severe	Extreme or cannot do
S12	Your day-to-day work?	None	Mild	Moderate	Severe	Extreme or cannot do

H1	Overall, in the past 30 days, how many days were these difficulties present?	*Record number of days* ____
H2	In the past 30 days, for how many days were you totally unable to carry out your usual activities or work because of any health condition?	*Record number of days* ____
H3	In the past 30 days, not counting the days that you were totally unable, for how many days did you cut back or reduce your usual activities or work because of any health condition?	*Record number of days* ____

This completes the questionnaire. Thank you.

WHODAS 2.0

WORLD **H**EALTH **O**RGANIZATION
DISABILITY **A**SSESSMENT **S**CHEDULE 2.0

12-item version, proxy-administered

This questionnaire asks about <u>difficulties due to health conditions</u> experienced by the person about whom you are responding in your role as friend, relative or carer. Health conditions include diseases or illnesses, other health problems that may be short or long lasting, injuries, mental or emotional problems, and problems with alcohol or drugs.

Think back over the <u>past 30 days</u> and, to the best of your knowledge, answer these questions thinking about how much difficulty your <u>friend, relative or carer</u> had while doing the following activities. (Note: the questionnaire uses the term "relative" to mean "friend", "relative" or "carer".) For each question, please circle only <u>one</u> response.

H4[a]	I am the _____ (choose one) of this person.	1 =	husband or wife	5 =	other relative
		2 =	parent	6 =	friend
		3 =	son or daughter	7 =	professional carer
		4 =	brother or sister	8 =	other (specify) _____

[a] Questions H1–H3 appear at the end of the questionnaire.

In the past 30 days, how much difficulty did your relative have in:						
S1	Standing for <u>long periods</u> such as <u>30 minutes</u>?	None	Mild	Moderate	Severe	Extreme or cannot do
S2	Taking care of his or her <u>household responsibilities</u>?	None	Mild	Moderate	Severe	Extreme or cannot do
S3	<u>Learning</u> a <u>new task</u>, for example, learning how to get to a new place?	None	Mild	Moderate	Severe	Extreme or cannot do
S4	How much of a problem did your relative have <u>joining in community activities</u> (for example, festivities, religious or other activities) in the same way as anyone else can?	None	Mild	Moderate	Severe	Extreme or cannot do
S5	How much has <u>your relative</u> been <u>emotionally affected</u> by his or her health condition?	None	Mild	Moderate	Severe	Extreme or cannot do

Please continue to next page...

In the past 30 days, how much difficulty did your relative have in:						
S6	Concentrating on doing something for ten minutes?	None	Mild	Moderate	Severe	Extreme or cannot do
S7	Walking a long distance such as a kilometre [or equivalent]?	None	Mild	Moderate	Severe	Extreme or cannot do
S8	Washing his or her whole body?	None	Mild	Moderate	Severe	Extreme or cannot do
S9	Getting dressed?	None	Mild	Moderate	Severe	Extreme or cannot do
S10	Dealing with people he or she does not know?	None	Mild	Moderate	Severe	Extreme or cannot do
S11	Maintaining a friendship?	None	Mild	Moderate	Severe	Extreme or cannot do
S12	His or her day-to-day work?	None	Mild	Moderate	Severe	Extreme or cannot do

H1	Overall, in the past 30 days, how many days were these difficulties present?	*Record number of days* ____
H2	In the past 30 days, for how many days were you totally unable to carry out your usual activities or work because of any health condition?	*Record number of days* ____
H3	In the past 30 days, not counting the days that you were totally unable, for how many days did you cut back or reduce your usual activities or work because of any health condition?	*Record number of days* ____

This completes the questionnaire. Thank you.

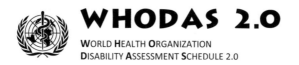

WHODAS 2.0
WORLD **H**EALTH **O**RGANIZATION
DISABILITY **A**SSESSMENT **S**CHEDULE 2.0

12+24-item version, interviewer-administered

Introduction

This instrument was developed by the WHO *Classification, Terminology and Standards* team, within the framework of the WHO/National Institutes of Health (NIH) Joint Project on Assessment and Classification of Disability.

Before using this instrument, interviewers must be trained using the manual *Measuring Health and Disability: Manual for WHO Disability Assessment Schedule – WHODAS 2.0* (WHO, 2010), which includes an interview guide and other training material.

The versions of the interview available are as follows:

- 36-item – Interviewer-administered[a]
- 36-item – Self-administered
- 36-item – Proxy-administered[b]
- 12-item – Interviewer-administered[c]
- 12-item – Self-administered
- 12-item – Proxy-administered
- 12+24-item – Interviewer-administered

   [a] A computerized version of the interview (*iShell*) is available for computer-assisted interviews or for data entry

   [b] Relatives, friends or caretakers

   [c] The 12-item version explains 81% of the variance of the more detailed 36-item version

For more details of the versions please refer to the WHODAS 2.0 manual *Measuring Health and Disability: Manual for WHO Disability Assessment Schedule – WHODAS 2.0* (WHO, 2010).

Permission to translate this instrument into any language should be obtained from WHO, and all translations should be prepared according to the WHO translation guidelines, as detailed in the accompanying manual.

For additional information, please visit www.who.int/whodas or contact:

Dr T Bedirhan Üstün
Classification, Terminology and Standards
Health Statistics and Informatics
World Health Organization (WHO)
1211 Geneva 27
Switzerland

Tel: + 41 22 791 3609
E-mail:ustunb@who.int

WHODAS 2.0

WORLD **H**EALTH **O**RGANIZATION
DISABILITY **A**SSESSMENT **S**CHEDULE 2.0

This questionnaire contains the interviewer-administered 12-item version of WHODAS 2.0.

Instructions to the interviewer are written in bold and italics – do not read these aloud

Text for the respondent to hear is written in

standard print in blue.

Read this text aloud

Section 1 Face sheet

Complete items F1–F5 before starting each interview				
F1	Respondent identity number			
F2	Interviewer identity number			
F3	Assessment time point (1, 2, etc)			
F4	Interview date	_____ day	_____ month	_____ year
F5	Living situation at time of interview (circle only one)	Independent in community		1
		Assisted living		2
		Hospitalized		3

Please continue to next page...

WHODAS 2.0

WORLD HEALTH ORGANIZATION
DISABILITY ASSESSMENT SCHEDULE 2.0

Section 2 Demographic and background information

This interview has been developed by the World Health Organization (WHO) to better understand the difficulties people may have due to their health conditions. The information that you provide in this interview is confidential and will be used only for research. The interview will take 10–20 minutes to complete.

For respondents from the general population (not the clinical population) say:

Even if you are healthy and have no difficulties, I need to ask all of the questions so that the survey is complete.

I will start with some background questions.

A1	**Record sex as observed**	Female	1
		Male	2
A2	How old are you now?	_____ years	
A3	How many years in all did you spend <u>studying in school, college or university</u>?	_____ years	
A4	What is your <u>current marital status</u>? **(Select the single best option)**	Never married	1
		Currently married	2
		Separated	3
		Divorced	4
		Widowed	5
		Cohabiting	6
A5	Which describes your <u>main work status</u> best? **(Select the single best option)**	Paid work	1
		Self employed, such as own your business or farming	2
		Non-paid work, such as volunteer or charity	3
		Student	4
		Keeping house/ homemaker	5
		Retired	6
		Unemployed (health reasons)	7
		Un employed (other reasons)	8
		Other (specify)_____ _____	9

Please continue to next page...

Section 3   Preamble

Say to respondent:

The interview is about difficulties people have because of health conditions.

Hand flashcard #1 to respondent

By health condition, I mean diseases or illnesses, or other health problems that may be short or long lasting; injuries; mental or emotional problems; and problems with alcohol or drugs.

Remember to keep all of your health problems in mind as you answer the questions. When I ask you about difficulties in doing an activity think about:

Point to flashcard #1 and explain that "difficulty with an activity" means:

- Increased effort
- Discomfort or pain
- Slowness
- Changes in the way you do the activity.

Say to respondent:

When answering, I'd like you to think back over the past 30 days. I would also like you to answer these questions thinking about how much difficulty you have had, on average, over the past 30 days, while doing the activity as you <u>usually</u> do it.

Hand flashcard #2 to respondent and say:

Use this scale when responding.

Read the scale aloud:

None, mild, moderate, severe, extreme or cannot do.

Ensure that the respondent can easily see flashcards #1 and #2 throughout the interview

Please continue to next page...

Section 4   Core questions

Show flashcard #2

In the past 30 days, how much difficulty did you have in:	None	Mild	Moderate	Severe	Extreme or cannot do
S1	Standing for long periods such as 30 minutes?	1	2	3	4	5
S2	Taking care of your household responsibilities?	1	2	3	4	5
S3	Learning a new task, for example, learning how to get to a new place?	1	2	3	4	5
S4	Joining in community activities (for example, festivities, religious or other activities) in the same way as anyone else can?	1	2	3	4	5
S5	How much have you been emotionally affected by your health problems?	1	2	3	4	5

If any of S1–S5 are endorsed (rated greater than none), continue with S6–S12. Otherwise, this is the end of the interview, in which case say:

This concludes our interview. Thank you for participating.

In the past 30 days, how much difficulty did you have in:	None	Mild	Moderate	Severe	Extreme or cannot do
S6	Concentrating on doing something for ten minutes?	1	2	3	4	5
S7	Walking a long distance such as a kilometre [or equivalent]?	1	2	3	4	5
S8	Washing your whole body?	1	2	3	4	5
S9	Getting dressed?	1	2	3	4	5
S10	Dealing with people you do not know?	1	2	3	4	5
S11	Maintaining a friendship?	1	2	3	4	5
S12	Your day-to-day work?	1	2	3	4	5

Please continue to next page...

Continue by administering the specified domains as follows:

If question is endorsed (coded 2–5)	Go to	Domain number
S3 or S6	⟹	1 on page 6
S1 or S7	⟹	2 on page 7
S8 or S9	⟹	3 on page 7
S10 or S11	⟹	4 on page 7
S2 or S12	⟹	5 on pages 8–9
S4 or S5	⟹	6 on page 10

Domain 1   Cognition

I am now going to ask some questions about <u>understanding and communicating</u>.

Show flashcards #1 and #2

In the past 30 days, how much difficulty did you have in:		None	Mild	Moderate	Severe	Extreme or cannot do
D1.2	<u>Remembering</u> to do <u>important things</u>?	1	2	3	4	5
D1.3	<u>Analysing and finding solutions to problems</u> in day-to-day life?	1	2	3	4	5
D1.5	<u>Generally understanding</u> what people say?	1	2	3	4	5
D1.6	<u>Starting and maintaining a conversation</u>?	1	2	3	4	5

Please continue to next page...

Domain 2   Mobility

I am now going to ask you about difficulties in <u>getting around</u>.

Show flashcards #1 and #2

In the past 30 days, how much difficulty did you have in:		None	Mild	Moderate	Severe	Extreme or cannot do
D2.2	<u>Standing up</u> from sitting down?	1	2	3	4	5
D2.3	<u>Moving</u> around <u>inside your home</u>?	1	2	3	4	5
D2.4	<u>Getting out</u> of your <u>home</u>?	1	2	3	4	5

Domain 3   Self-care

I am now going to ask you about difficulties in <u>taking care of yourself</u>.

Show flashcards #1 and #2

In the past 30 days, how much difficulty did you have in:		None	Mild	Moderate	Severe	Extreme or cannot do
D3.3	<u>Eating</u>?	1	2	3	4	5
D3.4	Staying <u>by yourself</u> for a <u>few days</u>?	1	2	3	4	5

Domain 4   Getting along

I am now going to ask you about difficulties in <u>getting along with people</u>. Please remember that I am asking only about difficulties that are due to health problems. By this I mean diseases or illnesses, injuries, mental or emotional problems and problems with alcohol or drugs.

Show flashcards #1 and #2

In the past 30 days, how much difficulty did you have in:		None	Mild	Moderate	Severe	Extreme or cannot do
D4.3	<u>Getting along</u> with people who are <u>close</u> to you?	1	2	3	4	5
D4.4	<u>Making new friends</u>?	1	2	3	4	5
D4.5	<u>Sexual activities</u>?	1	2	3	4	5

Please continue to next page...

Domain 5   Life activities

5(1)   Household activities

I am now going to ask you about activities involved in maintaining your household, and in caring for the people who you live with or are close to. These activities include cooking, cleaning, shopping, caring for others and caring for your belongings.

Show flashcards #1 and #2.

Because of your health condition, in the past 30 days, how much difficulty did you have in:	**None**	**Mild**	**Moderate**	**Severe**	**Extreme or cannot do**
D5.2 Doing your most important household tasks <u>well</u>?	1	2	3	4	5
D5.3 Getting all the household work <u>done</u> that you needed to do?	1	2	3	4	5
D5.4 Getting your household work done as <u>quickly</u> as needed?	1	2	3	4	5

If any of the responses to D5.2–D5.4 are rated greater than none (coded as "1"), ask:

D5.01	In the past 30 days, on how many days did you reduce or completely miss <u>household work</u> because of your health condition?	*Record number of days* ____

If respondent works (paid, non-paid, self-employed) or goes to school, complete questions D5.6–D5.10 on the next page. Otherwise, skip to D6.2 on page 10.

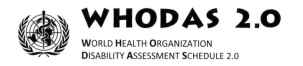
5(2)   Work or school activities

Now I will ask some questions about your work or school activities.

Show flashcards #1 and #2

Because of your health condition, in the past 30 days how much difficulty did you have in:	None	Mild	Moderate	Severe	Extreme or cannot do
D5.6 Doing your most important work/school tasks <u>well</u>?	1	2	3	4	5
D5.7 Getting all the work <u>done</u> that you need to do?	1	2	3	4	5
D5.8 Getting your work done as <u>quickly</u> as needed?	1	2	3	4	5
D5.9 Have you had to work at a <u>lower level</u> because of a health condition?				No	1
				Yes	2
D5.10 Did you <u>earn less money</u> as the result of a health condition?				No	1
				Yes	2

If any of D5.6–D5.10 are rated greater than none (coded as "1"), ask:

D5.02	In the past 30 days, on how many days did you <u>miss work for half a day or more</u> because of your health condition?	***Record number of days*** ____

Please continue to next page...

Domain 6   Participation

Now, I am going to ask you about your participation in society and the impact of your health problems on you and your family. Some of these questions may involve problems that go beyond the past 30 days; however, in answering, please focus on the past 30 days. Again, remember to answer these questions while thinking about your health problems: physical, mental or emotional, alcohol or drug related.

Show flashcards #1 and #2

In the past 30 days:		None	Mild	Moderate	Severe	Extreme or cannot do
D6.2	How much of a problem did you have because of barriers or hindrances in the world around you?	1	2	3	4	5
D6.3	How much of a problem did you have living with dignity because of the attitudes and actions of others?	1	2	3	4	5
D6.4	How much time did you spend on your health condition, or its consequences?	1	2	3	4	5
D6.6	How much has your health been a drain on the financial resources of you or your family?	1	2	3	4	5
D6.7	How much of a problem did your family have because of your health problems?	1	2	3	4	5
D6.8	How much of a problem did you have in doing things by yourself for relaxation or pleasure?	1	2	3	4	5

H1	Overall, in the past 30 days, <u>how many days</u> were these difficulties present?	*Record number of days* ____
H2	In the past 30 days, for how many days were you <u>totally unable</u> to carry out your usual activities or work because of any health condition?	*Record number of days* ____
H3	In the past 30 days, not counting the days that you were totally unable, for how many days did you <u>cut back</u> or <u>reduce</u> your usual activities or work because of any health condition?	*Record number of days* ____

This concludes our interview. Thank you for participating.

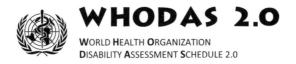

WHODAS 2.0
WORLD HEALTH ORGANIZATION
DISABILITY ASSESSMENT SCHEDULE 2.0

Health conditions:

- Diseases, illnesses or other health problems
- Injuries
- Mental or emotional problems
- Problems with alcohol
- Problems with drugs

Having difficulty with an activity means:

- Increased effort
- Discomfort or pain
- Slowness
- Changes in the way you do the activity

Think about the past 30 days only.

WHODAS 2.0

WORLD HEALTH ORGANIZATION
DISABILITY ASSESSMENT SCHEDULE 2.0

Flashcard 2

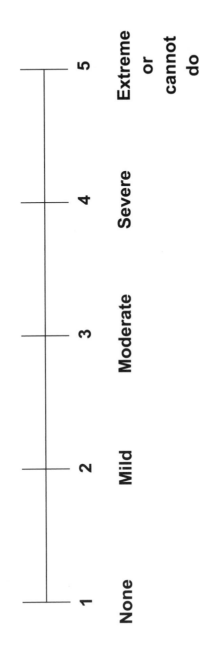

1	2	3	4	5
None	Mild	Moderate	Severe	Extreme or cannot do